An Introduction to
Paediatric Neurology

An Introduction to Paediatric Neurology

GWILYM HOSKING

MB, MRCP, DCH

Consultant Paediatric Neurologist
The Ryegate Centre and
The Children's Hospital, Sheffield

faber and faber

First published in 1982
by Faber & Faber Limited
3 Queen Square London WC1
Set, printed and bound in Great Britain by
Fakenham Press Limited
Fakenham Norfolk
All rights reserved

British Library Cataloguing in Publication Data

Hosking, Gwilym
  An introduction to paediatric neurology
  1. Paediatric neurology
  I. Title
  618.92'8   RJ486

  ISBN 0–571–11848–8
  ISBN 0–571–11849–6 Pbk

PARENTS

My own parents

Henry Thomas, Friend, Farmer and Father-in-Law

Contents

NEOPLASTIC DISEASE OF THE NERVOUS SYSTEM

COMMON NEUROLOGICAL SYMPTOMS

Illustrations

Preface

Neurological disorders in children are common. They range from migraine and epilepsy to a variety of neuromuscular problems, to mental retardation and the rare neurodegenerative diseases.

While children with a possible neurological dysfunction demand careful and skilful medical evaluation they also require care and support from a number of the other professional groups. These range from the medical and nursing to the professions allied to medicine, education and social work.

Without some knowledge of the underlying physical basis of children with neurological or developmental abnormalities, care is inevitably more difficult to provide. This book attempts to fill in what, for some, may be a gap in their knowledge.

The medical aspect of childhood neurological handicap is presented in the hope that the information contained will enhance the relevant caring professions' ability to help, support and educate the children in question. While it is not a book written for doctors, it may, nevertheless, be found useful by them.

As the readers are likely to vary greatly in the extent of their medical knowledge the book contains at the beginning a glossary of terms followed by two explanatory chapters; one giving a series of simple anatomical drawings while the second attempts to describe and explain the procedures that are commonly applied in the investigation and evaluation of children with possible neurological disease.

Throughout the book an attempt is made to emphasise the need for a team approach to any child suffering from any of the conditions which are described.

Acknowledgements

Few authors are able to produce texts entirely by themselves, but may do so with the help of others: I am indebted to many.

I am confident that the artistic skills of Mrs Audrey Besterman seen in Chapter 2 will enable many to understand more easily the complexities of neuro-anatomy.

I am grateful to Dr Norman Lewtas for Figures 3/4, 3/5, 3/6, 3/7, and 3/8 and to Dr Tom Powell for his description of the principles of CAT scanning in Chapter 3.

Figures 8/1, 8/2, 14/1, and 15/1 first appeared in articles in the *Nursing Mirror* during March and April 1979. I thank the Editor, *Nursing Mirror*, for permission to reproduce them.

Mr Tony Potter of the Department of Human Genetics, the University of Sheffield kindly provided the karyotypes in Chapter 6 and for these I am most grateful.

Throughout the remainder of the text the illustrations that appear are as the result of advice and support of Mrs Dorothy Huntingdon, the Department of Medical Illustration, Sheffield Area Health Authority, to whom I extend my appreciation and thanks.

It is my colleagues in the various professions at the Ryegate Centre that I most acknowledge and thank for their advice and inspiration. It is my privilege and pleasure to work with a well-knit team of dedicated professionals willing to share their skills on the understanding that by so doing it will be to the advantage of the child who is being described within this book. It is for them and other similarly dedicated persons that I write.

In conclusion I would like to single out two persons who have, above all others, made the production of this book possible. Mrs Janet Chapman has typed numerous drafts with patient skill and with speed; for this I am most grateful. My sincere thanks are also due to Dr Gillian Maddocks who has provided helpful and constructive criticism of the book throughout its writing.

Although I have received much help with the production of this book the responsibility for the accuracy of the facts and the opinions expressed rest entirely with me.

G.H., 1981

Glossary

acid-base disturbances   Disturbances of the acidity or alkalinity of the body fluids

acidosis   Body fluids are more acid than normal

adducted   Moved towards the mid line of the body

adhesions   The sticking together of two parts or surfaces—often following an inflammatory process, e.g. intestines

aetiology   The cause of

agenesis   Failure to develop

amino acid   Proteins are made up of amino acids which are nitrogen containing organic acids

amnesia   Loss of memory

amplitude   Measure of the strength of an electrical current

amplification   To make larger; to increase the size of

anaemia   Reduction in the blood cells or the amount of haemoglobin in the blood cells so reducing the oxygen carrying potential of the blood

anoxia   Shortage of oxygen

anterior   In front of—opposite of posterior

antibiotic (antimicrobial)   A drug which prevents organisms multiplying

antibody   A protein produced by the body as a defence mechanism, which is able to neutralise the corresponding antigen

antigen   A protein not normally present in the body that will induce the production of antibody

aorta   The large artery which leads out of the left side of the heart

aphasia   Without speech

apnoea   Absence of spontaneous breathing

artery   A blood vessel that leads blood away from the heart

arthritis   Inflammation of joints

articulation   Production of speech using the muscles of the mouth and tongue

asymptomatic   No symptoms

atrophy   Wasting, particularly of muscle

autopsy   Examination of a body after death

benign   Non-malignant

bimanual   Two handed

biochemical   Chemicals associated with the function of the body

biopsy   Removal of a small amount of body tissue in order to confirm or make a diagnosis

blood levels   The amount of a certain substance in the blood

buccal   In the mouth, particularly the inside of the cheek

bulbar paresis   Paralysis of the muscles in the throat which control swallowing

calcification   The accumulation of calcium deposits

capillary   The small blood vessels that connect arteries to veins

carbohydrate   A sugar or a starch

cardiomyopathy   Disease of the heart muscle not caused by specific infection

cardiovascular   Concerning the heart and circulatory system

cataracts   Opacities of the lens of the eye causing varying degrees of visual impairment

catheter   Tube used to remove fluids, e.g. blood, urine

cerebral   Concerning the brain

cervical vertebrae   The small bones in the neck which form part of the spine

chelating agent   A substance which combines with metals

chemotherapy   Use of drugs as treatment

chorea   Irregular involuntary movements of the limbs

chromatography   A technique for separating the constituents of a mixture

cirrhosis   Damage to the liver

coma   Insensibility, sleep, stupor

complement A protein which takes part in the reaction between antigens and antibodies

concussion Interruption of the function of the brain as a result of a blow to the head

conduction The passage of an impulse along a nerve

congenital Existing at birth

contractures Permanent contraction because of inelastic fibrous tissue formation

cryptorchidism Failure of testes to descend into the scrotum

cubitus valgus The forearm is angled out from the elbow, so giving a wide angle

cutaneous Pertaining to the skin

decerebrate Functioning without higher cortical activity. No consciousness; breathing and cardiac function only

demyelination The destruction and loss of the myelin sheath around nerve fibres

depigmentation Loss of skin pigment

dermatoglyphics Study of skin ridge patterns

diaphragmatic Concerned with the diaphragm (the muscular septum separating chest and abdomen)

distal Away from the centre

effusion Collection of fluid in a serous cavity, e.g. pleural or peritoneal cavity

elongation The process of making something longer

embolus Obstructing a blood vessel by particulate bodies—blood clot, fat, air or other objects

embryology Science of the development of the embryo (or fetus)

endocrine The ductless glands that secrete into the bloodstream. Examples include adrenals, thyroid, parathyroid, pituitary, pancreas, ovaries

enzyme Protein that acts as a catalyst

epicanthic folds Projection of nasal fold to the eyelid

exanthem A disease accompanied by a specific rash

exchange transfusion Transfusion in the newborn in which a large proportion of the blood volume is gradually replaced over about two hours by donor blood. This has been most commonly used in the treatment of Rhesus babies

extensor A muscle which extends or straightens a part

fasciculation Minute spontaneous contractions of small muscle fibres

fatty infiltration Infiltration of tissue with fat

febrile Related to a fever

fertilised Union of male and female germ cells whereby reproduction takes place

fibroblasts Branched cells found throughout connective tissue which synthesise collagen and elastin

fibromata Benign tumours of connective tissue

flexion Being bent—opposite to extension

fetus (foetus) Unborn child

fontanelle Soft spot in the infant skull before it has fully fused

fracture A break in a bone

fundus (optic) Back part of the eye ball through which the optic nerve enters

gait Manner of walking and running

gastro-enteritis Inflammation of the stomach and intestines

gastro-intestinal tract The gut; including the mouth, oesophagus, stomach, small and large intestines, rectum and anus

genitalia The sex organs

genito-urinary system Reproductive (sex) and urinary organs

glial Relating to neuroglia tissue (brain cells) of the brain

glucose A sugar

gynaecomastia Over-development of the male breast

gyrus of brain Folds in the white matter of the brain separated by fissures or sulci

hamstring muscles Group of muscles at the back of thighs

haemangioma Structural abnormality of blood vessels

haematoma A large clot of blood in a tissue or body part

haemorrhage Bleeding

hemiplegia   Paralysis of one side of the body

hemispherectomy   The surgical removal of one complete cerebral hemisphere

hepatosplenomegaly   Enlargement of the liver and spleen

herpetic   A skin lesion with small vesicles due to infection with the virus, herpes simplex

heterozygotes   Individuals that have two differing genes in a corresponding part (or locus) of a pair of chromosomes

homozygotes   Having the same gene in the corresponding locus of the pair of chromosomes

hydramnios   Excessive amniotic fluid in the uterus (or womb)

hyperbilirubinaemia   High level of the bile pigment—bilirubin—in the blood. This causes jaundice

hypercalcaemia   High level of calcium in the blood. (Hypocalcaemia = low level)

hypernatraemia   High level of sodium in the blood (Hyponatraemia = low level)

hyperteliorism (ocular)   Abnormally widely spaced eyes

hypertension   High blood pressure (Hypotension = low blood pressure)

hyperuricaemia   High level of uric acid in the blood

hypoglycaemia   Low level of sugar in the blood

hypomagnesaemia   Low level of magnesium in the blood

hypothermia   Low body temperature

hypotonic   Low muscle tone—floppy

hypoxia   Diminished amount of available oxygen

iatrogenic   Doctor induced

ictal   A seizure; post-ictal—after a seizure

immunisation   The production of some immunity from disease by stimulating the body's own defence

inborn errors of metabolism   An abnormality of some aspects of the body's metabolism due to a congenital defect of an enzyme system

incidence   The number of cases of a disorder in a certain number of births

incontinence   Failure to control urinary and/or faecal voiding

infarction   Death of tissue due to the stoppage of its blood supply

inflammation   The response of tissue to injury by trauma or infection

inoculation   Introduction of infectious material into a culture medium to produce growth and subsequent identification of the bacteria and antibiotic sensitivities

intercostal   Between two ribs

intervertebral disc   The disc between two vertebrae

intracellular   Inside a body cell

intracerebral   Inside the brain

intracranial   Inside the head

intraneuronal   Inside a nerve

intra-uterine (in utero)   Inside the uterus

intravenous   Into a vein

intrinsic   From within

insidious   Slow in onset

involuntary   Not under voluntary control

iris   Pigmented membrane behind the cornea of the eye, perforated by the pupil

ischaemia   Local and temporary deficiency of blood supply

isotope   A chemical element having the same atomic number as another but a different number of neutrons

jaundice   Yellowness of skin due to an excessive amount of bile pigment in the blood and body (see hyperbilirubinaemia)

kypho-scoliosis   Abnormal curvature of the spine forwards and sideways

kyphosis   Abnormal curvature of the spine forwards

lactose   A sugar derived from milk

laxative   A medication which promotes evacuation of the bowels

lesion   The site of structural or functional change in body tissue produced by disease or injury

lethal   Causes death

lethargy   Stupor or profound drowsiness

light microscope   A microscope producing magnification of particles from about ten times to one hundred times their size, and containing a light source

linear fracture Fracture along the length of a bone

lipid A fat or fat ester

lipoprotein Compound of a fat and protein

liquor amni The fluid in the cavity of the uterus that surrounds the fetus

litigation Taking legal action

liver A large organ situated in the upper part of the abdomen on the right

lobar pneumonia Pneumonia affecting a lobe(s) of a lung

lumbar vertebrae The spine between the thorax and sacrum

lymphadenopathy Enlargement of lymph glands

macula (of eye) A light sensitive area on the retina of the eye

malformation Defective formation

marrow Soft material filling cavities in bone

mass lesion A lesion in which there is some structural change; also, cause-effects due to the size of the lesion or mass

maternal Pertaining to the female parent

micromelia Abnormal smallness of hands or feet

micropsia Defective vision with objects seeming smaller than usual

micturition Discharging urine from the bladder: urination

morbidity The effects of an illness on living

morphology The study of structure

mortality Death—the frequency of death in a certain community or caused by certain diseases

multifactorial Due to more than one factor

murmur A sound heard with a stethoscope over large vessels of the heart, suggesting an abnormality of blood flow

mutism Inability to speak

myelin A soft material surrounding the axons of some nerves

myelitis Inflammation of the spinal cord

necrotic Death of tissue

neonatal The first month of life

neoplasm (neoplastic)   New growth (tumours—benign and malignant)

nephritis   Inflammation of kidney

neuronal plexus   Collection of nerves

neurophysiological   Related to the physiology of the nervous system

obesity   An excessive accumulation of fat in the body

oedema   An abnormal accumulation of fluid in intercellular spaces of the body

operative   By operation

opisthotonic posturing   Spasm in which the head, spine and hands (and feet) extend backwards in an arch

ophthalmoplegia   Paralysis of eye movements

ophthalmoscope   An instrument for examining the interior of the eye

optic chiasm   Crossing over of optic nerves and tracts

optic nerve   Nerve from the back of the eye to the optic chiasm

oral   Pertaining to the mouth

orthopaedics   Concerning all aspects of the musculo-skeletal system including development, disease and treatment

osteoporosis   Thinning of the bone

otitis media   Infection or inflammation of the middle ear cavity

otorrhoea   Discharge from the ear

ovaries   Female reproductive glands close to the uterus

ovum   The female reproductive cell

papilloedema   Oedema and swelling of the optic nerve

papilloma   Benign neoplasm of epithelial cells

paraplegia   Paralysis of both lower limbs

paraesthesia   Disordered sensation such as tingling and pins and needles

paresis   Slight or incomplete paralysis

paroxysmal   Sudden temporary attack

pellagra   Syndrome caused by deficiency of nicotinic acid characterised by dementia and diarrhoea

perinatal   During the first week of life

peripheral   On the outside or away from the centre

peritoneal dialysis Changing the chemicals in the body by instilling through a needle into the peritoneal cavity a special solution. After a short interval this fluid is then drained off again. The process is repeated a number of times

peroneal group of muscles A group of muscles on the outer side of the leg between the knee and the foot

petechiae Small red spots on the skin formed by effusion of blood

pharyngitis Inflammation of the pharynx (or throat)

photophobia Intolerance of light

physiotherapy Therapy by physical means

platelets Blood cells concerned with the clotting of blood

plexus A network of vessels or nerves

polycythaemia Increase in the number of red blood cells in the circulation

polycystic Composed of many cysts

polydactyly Presence of supernumerary fingers or toes

polymorphonuclear leucocytes Many nuclei of various shapes. The most common form of white blood cells

posterior Behind—opposite of anterior

post-traumatic Following trauma or physical accident

posture Relating to position

premature Born before expected—before the 38th week of pregnancy

prenatal Before birth

prevalence Number of cases of a disorder in a specific age group within a population or the number of cases in a population

primitive reflexes Automatic neurological reflexes normally only seen in the developing infant

prognosis Outlook

prone Lying face down

prophylaxis Prevention of disease

proprioceptive disorders Disorders affecting sense of position and certain aspects of fine touch

proptosis Protrusion of eyeballs

proximal   Near to the centre

psychologist   Studies intellectual and behavioural patterns

psychometry   Measurement of intellectual function

ptosis   Dropping of eyelid(s)

puberty   Onset of sexual (and other) adult characteristics

pupil   The centre of the eye through which light passes

pus   Dead white cells and tissue exudate

pyrexia   Fever—elevated body temperature

quadriparesis   Weakness of all four limbs

quadriplegia   Paralysis of all four limbs

radiotherapy   Treatment with x-ray or radioactive substances

recanalisation   Re-establishing a tract or canal—usually a blood vessel

reflex activity   Automatic response to a given stimulus

refractive disorders   Visual disorders due to an optic defect in the eye, i.e. cornea, the lens or the shape of the eye

re-innervation   Nerves regrowing into muscles

renal   Concerning the kidney

resection   Remove surgically

respiratory arrest   Breathing stopped

retinitis   Inflammation or degeneration of the retina of the back of the eye

retrograde   Backwards

rhinorrhoea   Discharge from the nose

sacral spine   Lower end of the spinal column

scoliosis   Curve of the spine to one side

scotoma   An area of blindness within the field of vision

scrotum   Sac containing the male testes

secondary (as in cancer)   A cancer deposit distant from the primary malignant cancer or tumour

seizure   Fit or convulsion

septic   Infected

septicaemia   An infection of the blood

serous otitis media   Sterile fluid in the middle ear cavity (glue ear)

siblings   Brothers and sisters

sinus An abnormal tract running from one body surface to another *or* a cavity in the skull or facial bones

slit lamp A light for the close examination of the front of the eye

solute A chemical that has been dissolved

spatula Flat, flexible, blunt knife or wooden blade used for either spreading ointments *or* for examining the mouth by depressing the tongue

spinal column The whole vertebral column or backbone

spleen Large rounded organ under the ribs on the left

squint When the eyes do not look in exactly the same direction—cross-eyed

startle reaction Reflex movement in response to various stimuli—often sound, vibration or sudden movement

stature Size, particularly height

stenosis Narrowing of a canal or tube

stereotactic surgery Operations deep in the brain in which small lesions are caused by the end of a probe directed to an exact position

steroids A group of drugs with a principally anti-inflammatory action and having a wide range of applications

stigmata Signs

stupor Depressed level of consciousness—less depressed than coma

subcutaneous Under the skin

supine Lying face upwards. With the forearm it will be with the palm upwards

suppositories Small cones which are administered rectally; they contain a medicament in a base which is soluble at body temperature

suprasellar Above the dorsum sellae of the skull or above the pituitary fossa

sympathetic nerve chain A nerve chain running alongside the spine that gives branches which innervate the heart, gut, eyes, salivary glands, bladder and partly controls the blood to the skin and other organs. It is not under voluntary control and forms part of the autonomic nervous system

syncope   Fainting

syndactyly   Webbing of fingers or toes

systemic   As in disease—a generalised disease

tachycardia   Fast heart rate

talipes equinovarus   Club foot. A foot which is rotated inwards with the toes pointing downwards

tendon   A cord of fibrous tissue that connects a muscle into a bone

termination of pregnancy   Abortion that is produced medically

testes   The male sex glands

tetany   Spasms of the hands and feet due to either overbreathing or abnormalities of body calcium

threatened abortion   Miscarriage that may or may not occur

thrombosis   Coagulation of blood in blood vessels causing a blockage

titre   A standard of purity or strength

toxaemia   Toxins in the circulation

traction   Pulling. A method used to treat some fractures

transection   Cut across

transversely   Across

trauma   Injury

tremor   Involuntary trembling

trimester   Relating to pregnancy which is divided into thirds—1st, 2nd and 3rd trimesters

truncal   Of the body or trunk

tumour   A lump, but frequently referring to a growth or cancer

unilateral   One side

urinary stasis   Urine collected in the bladder and not being voided

uterus   Womb

varicella   Chicken pox

vascular   Concerning blood vessels

vasoconstriction   Constriction of blood vessels

vacuolated lymphocytes   White blood cells with cavities due to substances being accumulated

vacuum extraction   A method of delivering a baby with a suction cap attached to the scalp

vein   A vessel that returns blood towards the heart

velocity   Speed in a given direction

ventrosuspension   Holding a baby under the chest when he is face downwards

vertebrae   The bones of the spinal column

vertigo   Giddiness

virus   An organism that is very much smaller than a bacterium and can only survive inside another cell

visual acuity   The strength of vision

visual fields   The area over which there is vision

Further reference may be made to:

The Faber Pocket Medical Dictionary, 3rd edition, revised by Elizabeth Forsythe MRCS, LRCP, DPH, published by Faber and Faber, London and Boston

Dorland's Pocket Medical Dictionary, 22nd edition, published by W. B. Saunders Co, Philadelphia

1. The child with a neurological problem

The specialty of paediatric or child neurology is concerned with neurological disorders which may cause problems in childhood. Such disorders can be grouped in several ways. In this book they have been divided into five groups:

1. Those which result from abnormal development of the brain and spinal cord

2. Those which occur as a result of the influence of generalised disease

3. Those due to external influences

4. Neoplastic disease

5. Groups of disorders which are considered together because of their major presenting symptoms or problems.

THE MEDICAL APPROACH TO A CHILD WITH A POSSIBLE NEUROLOGICAL DISORDER

History taking

Doctors are taught to approach a diagnostic problem by first taking a detailed history and then conducting a systematic physical examination of the patient. A provisional diagnosis, or a list of possible diagnoses, is made as a result of the history, and the subsequent examination is expected to be confirmatory. Occasionally a 'spot diagnosis' can be made simply on the appearance of a child or after a minimal number of questions. However, taking a detailed and careful history from *all* patients and parents is recognised as being very important. Individual doctors develop a routine of history taking to avoid omitting relevant details. The problem of coping with anxious parents and often unco-operative children requires considerable adaptation and flexibility if a comprehensive history is to be taken.

The doctor should carefully elicit the family history. Knowledge of a previous occurrence within the family of the same or similar disorder not only provides information of the genetic inheritance but may help with the diagnosis. A dominantly inherited condition will often affect several members of a family because a single abnormal gene inherited from either parent will cause the condition; whereas a recessive condition requires two genes, one from each parent, neither of whom will themselves be affected. First-cousin marriages significantly increase the chances of a recessively inherited condition occurring. Certain disorders occur as a result of abnormal genes on the X chromosome. Females have two X chromosomes and so in the absence of two abnormal genes, one on each chromosome, the disorder is not apparent. However, males have only one X chromosome and an abnormal gene will manifest itself if present. Such conditions are, therefore, termed *X-linked recessive* disorders and well-known examples of these are the Duchenne type of muscular dystrophy and haemophilia. So the mother of a boy with an X-linked recessive condition may produce boys, half of whom will have the disorder because they have inherited the abnormal gene from their mother, and girls, half of whom turn out to be *carriers* like herself but in whom the condition is not manifest because of the presence of the second normal gene on the other chromosome. If the affected male is able to reproduce, all his daughters are likely to be carriers, but none of his sons will be affected because he passes his normal Y chromosome to his sons and his abnormal X chromosome to daughters.

With dominantly inherited conditions there is a 50 per cent chance of an offspring being affected because only one abnormal gene is required. In a recessively inherited condition there is not a high chance of an offspring being affected (except in a first-cousin marriage) because of the need to acquire an abnormal gene from each parent, but a 25 per cent chance of a sibling being similarly affected. Abnormal genes can arise without a family history; such a newly developed abnormal gene is called a *mutation*, and occurs when ovum and sperm are first fused. Such parents are not at risk of producing further abnormal children. Many genetically determined disorders, whether occurring as fresh mutations or as being dominantly inherited conditions, may be variably expressed (incomplete penetrance) producing varying degrees of disability or abnormality. The initial enquiry into the family history not only may enable or aid the diagnosis of a genetically determined disorder to be made, but precedes important genetic counselling which will ultimately need to be given.

Additionally, the family history should reveal whether there are any other medical or social problems which may be as relevant to the health and welfare of the patient as evidence suggesting a genetic disorder.

The history must include details of the pregnancy, delivery, and early neonatal period. Pregnancy is a time of rapid differentiation and growth from the fertilised ovum to the viable, healthy, newborn infant. Many factors can, and do, have a profound influence on the development of the fetus: these include maternal infections such as rubella, cytomegalovirus and, rarely, toxoplasmosis and syphilis; the smoking of cigarettes during pregnancy; and the taking of drugs whether given on medical advice or not.

Antepartum haemorrhage and pre-eclamptic toxaemia are causes for concern, since adequate nutrition of the fetus may be impaired by these and may give rise to developmental problems.

Reduced fetal movements are sometimes noted by mothers of children with severe congenital neuromuscular disorders. Hydramnios (excessive amniotic fluid) is encountered not only in association with oesophageal atresia but also with congenital dystrophia myotonica. Oligohydramnios (deficiency of amniotic fluid) has been associated by some in the aetiology of conditions such as talipes equinovarus (club foot).

Labour and delivery is a precarious time at which several events may prove to be hazardous to the infant. Prolonged rupture of the membranes, prolapsed cord, breech presentation, precipitate delivery, and delay in the onset of respiration are well-known problems which need to be dealt with rapidly and expertly to reduce the possibility of lasting ill effects to the infant. Unfortunately, this is not always the case and the occurrence of one of these complications may be relevant to neurological problems which the infant or child may later present.

Premature onset of labour may precede the problems so well recognised in the prematurely born—respiratory distress syndrome, hypothermia, hypoglycaemia, hyperbilirubinaemia, intra-ventricular haemorrhage, and infection. Although most of the problems of prematurity can be managed with careful and intensive neonatal care, prematurity is still, in some cases, associated with developmental delay and impaired neurological function.

The 'small for dates' infant who has suffered from intra-uterine malnutrition needs very careful nursing in the perinatal period, when pneumonia (inhalational during labour), hypothermia, and hypoglycaemia may be hazardous.

It is helpful to know something of the general state of the baby during the first few weeks of life. Tube feeding and hypotonia may be acceptable in the extremely premature, but in the full-term infant these may be suggestive of either significant neuromuscular disease, a more central 'brain damage', or a generally ill infant.

Seizures or fits in the newborn may be caused by several factors of which hypoglycaemia and hypocalcaemia are particularly common and treatable. If these are not the cause, then the underlying factor may be more sinister and relevant to the infant's future well-being and development.

The importance of a developmental history should be obvious. The taking of such a history may be very difficult, as parents seldom recollect 'milestones' accurately. Often to please the doctor they will guess at an answer or give what they feel is the 'correct' answer. The older the child, the less accurately will the milestones be recalled; but on the other hand, a detailed developmental history is not as important in the older child as in the younger child. The developmental history will often end up as an enquiry as to when the child first walked, talked, or used a potty; or as a suggested comparison with the early development of a sibling or other child.

A history of previous illnesses, operations, and immunisations should be obtained. The last part of the history is often the enquiry about the problems with which the child is currently being seen by the doctor. This will be combined with an enquiry about the current state of general health, physical and emotional, together with details of school progress when appropriate.

The details at this later part of the history will emerge in subsequent chapters and only a few general points need to be made here. The parents and the child need to be allowed, at least initially, to describe the problems as they see them, and only afterwards should they be guided into giving an accurate and ordered description. It is important not to ask questions that will direct the parents into giving a particular answer. However, the last part of the questioning may be used to ask several direct questions such as 'How is the hearing?', 'How is the balance?', or 'Does he have any headache?'

Any part of the history may be considerably enhanced by the inspection of reports from schools and clinics, and hospital case records.

Physical examination

A detailed examination is undertaken. This should be partly tailored by the knowledge gained from taking the history but must be complete and comprehensive. A formal examination as used with adults may be difficult in the very young child—the important factor is that the examiner must have some sort of order in his own mind. The examination should enable observations to be made of the child's behaviour, relationship with parents in the clinic setting, and current developmental status as well as the more physical aspects manifest in the general and neurological examination.

Even if there is maximum co-operation from a child for an examination, it is important not to over-interpret findings or the lack of them, but to be prepared to re-assess and re-examine. Naturally, such apparent procrastination is not advocated for acute conditions. More specific aspects of the examination will be dealt with in subsequent chapters, as will investigations that may need to be performed in children with neurological problems. It needs to be emphasised that no investigations should be considered routine, because many are unpleasant for children, time consuming, and expensive.

After the detailed history and examination it should be possible to make a diagnosis. A diagnosis may need confirming by further investigations. The doctor must then assess the significance of the disease or disorder to the child and the family. The short- and long-term management may then be discussed and genetic counselling undertaken if appropriate.

FURTHER READING

Emery, A. E. H. (1979). *Elements of Medical Genetics*, 5th edition. Churchill Livingstone, Edinburgh.

Forfar, J. O. and Arneil, G. C. (1978). *Textbook of Paediatrics*, 2nd edition. Churchill Livingstone, Edinburgh.

Illingworth, R. S. (1979). *The Normal Child*, 7th edition. Churchill Livingstone, Edinburgh.

Illingworth, R. S. (1980). *The Development of the Infant and Young Child*, 7th edition. Churchill Livingstone, Edinburgh.

Paine, R. S. and Oppe, T. E. (1971). *Neurological Examination of Children*. Spastics International Medical Publications. Clinics in Developmental Medicine No 20/21. William Heinemann Medical Books Ltd, London.

2. Basic anatomical illustrations

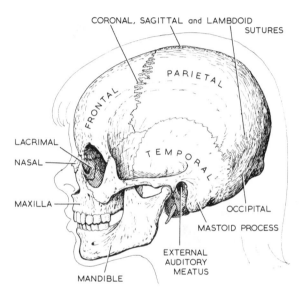

Fig. 2/1 Side view of the skull

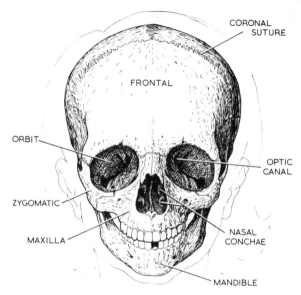

Fig. 2/2 Front view of the skull

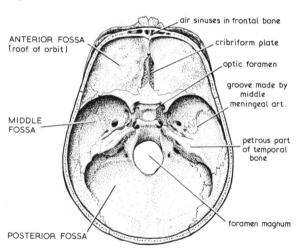

Fig. 2/3 Inside view of the skull

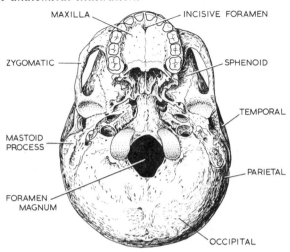

Fig. 2/4 Base of the skull

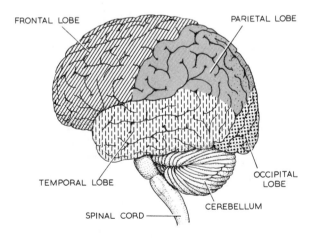

Fig. 2/5 Side view of the brain seen from the left

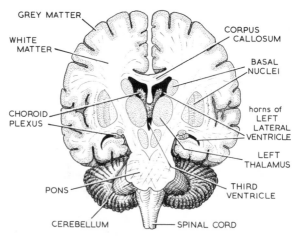

Fig. 2/6 Coronal section through cerebral hemispheres and brainstem, seen from the front

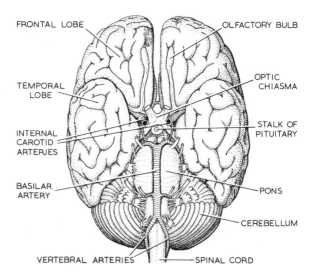

Fig. 2/7 The base of the brain showing the major arteries which form the circle of Willis

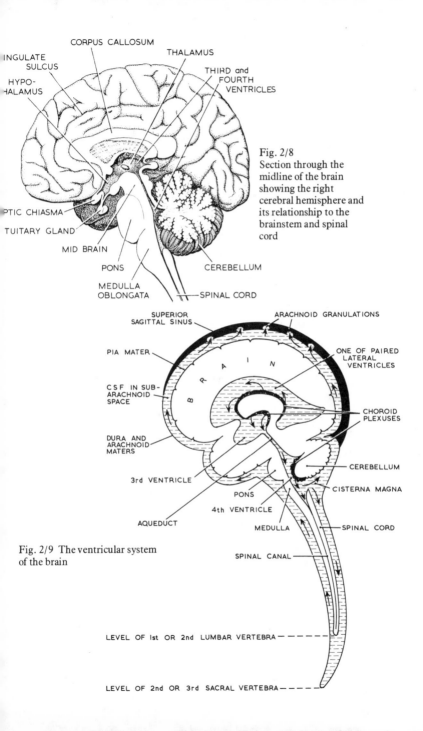

CORPUS CALLOSUM

CINGULATE
SULCUS

THALAMUS

HYPO-
THALAMUS

THIRD and
FOURTH
VENTRICLES

Fig. 2/8
Section through the
midline of the brain
showing the right
cerebral hemisphere and
its relationship to the
brainstem and spinal
cord

OPTIC CHIASMA

PITUITARY GLAND

MID BRAIN

PONS

CEREBELLUM

MEDULLA
OBLONGATA

SPINAL CORD

SUPERIOR
SAGITTAL SINUS

ARACHNOID GRANULATIONS

PIA MATER

ONE OF PAIRED
LATERAL
VENTRICLES

B R A I N

CSF IN SUB-
ARACHNOID
SPACE

CHOROID
PLEXUSES

DURA AND
ARACHNOID
MATERS

CEREBELLUM

3rd VENTRICLE

CISTERNA MAGNA

PONS

AQUEDUCT

4th VENTRICLE

MEDULLA

SPINAL CORD

SPINAL CANAL

Fig. 2/9 The ventricular system
of the brain

LEVEL OF 1st OR 2nd LUMBAR VERTEBRA

LEVEL OF 2nd OR 3rd SACRAL VERTEBRA

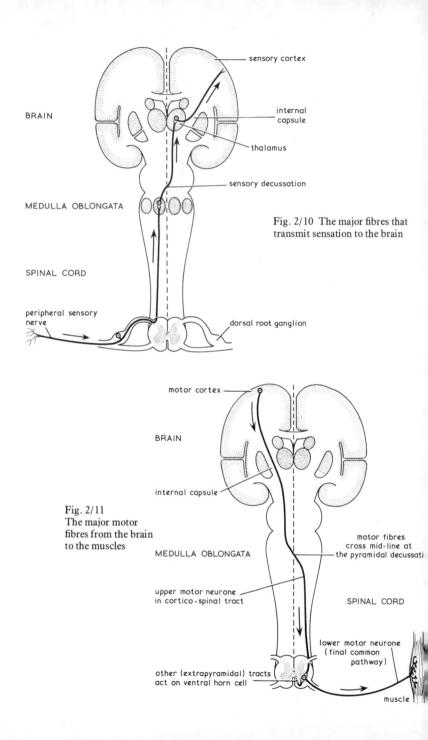

sensory cortex

internal capsule

BRAIN

thalamus

sensory decussation

MEDULLA OBLONGATA

Fig. 2/10 The major fibres that transmit sensation to the brain

SPINAL CORD

peripheral sensory nerve

dorsal root ganglion

motor cortex

BRAIN

internal capsule

Fig. 2/11
The major motor fibres from the brain to the muscles

MEDULLA OBLONGATA

motor fibres cross mid-line at the pyramidal decussati

upper motor neurone in cortico-spinal tract

SPINAL CORD

lower motor neurone (final common pathway)

other (extrapyramidal) tracts act on ventral horn cell

muscle

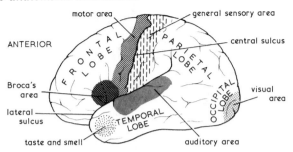

Fig. 2/12 Side view of the brain illustrating the major localisation of function

FURTHER READING

Gibson, J. (1978). *Human Biology: Elementary Anatomy and Physiology for Students and Nurses*, 3rd edition. Faber and Faber, London and Boston.

Grays Anatomy, 36th edition (1980). Longman Group Limited, Edinburgh.

Pearce, E. (1975). *Anatomy and Physiology for Nurses*, 16th edition. Faber and Faber, London and Boston.

Sears, W. G. and Winwood, R. S. (1974). *Anatomy and Physiology for Nurses and Students of Human Biology*, 5th edition. Edward Arnold (Publishers) Limited, London.

3. Common neurological investigations

PLAIN X-RAY STUDIES

Skull x-rays are taken for a variety of reasons. If a brain tumour is suspected it is sometimes possible to see evidence of its presence from either erosion of bone adjacent to the tumour or calcium within it. If the tumour is very large or interfering with the circulation of the cerebrospinal fluid (CSF) in the brain it may cause an increase in pressure in the head. Raised intra-cranial pressure, if it is of some duration, will be apparent on plain skull x-rays. Brain scars will sometimes contain calcium and this will be shown up on a simple x-ray. In the case of head injuries skull x-rays are almost a routine investigation in order to identify a possible fracture.

The technique of skull radiography is simple, with pictures usually taken from at least a side (lateral), front and basal view (Figs. 3/1a and b; 3/2a and b). For the child, the only need is to lie with the head in a particular position for a few seconds. Nevertheless due to the strangeness of the surroundings and the rather frightening appearance of the machines the younger child may need considerable reassurance.

X-ray of spine will be undertaken if there is a possibility of fracture or dislocation of the spine due to trauma; a suspicion of a tumour in or around the spinal column; or if a congenital structural abnormality is suspected.

In the child having the spine x-rayed the procedure will, in principle, be the same as for skull x-rays.

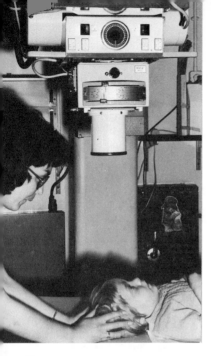

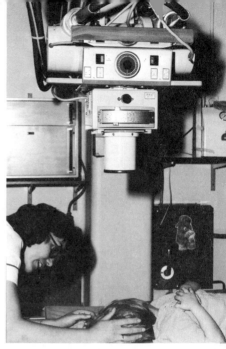

Fig. 3/1a Taking a skull x-ray
(front view)

Fig. 3/1b Taking a skull x-ray
(side view)

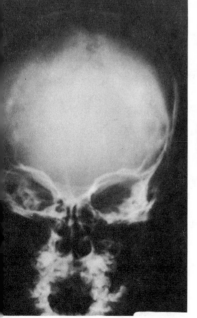

Fig. 3/2a (*left*) Skull x-ray from the
front)

Fig. 3/2b (*above*) Skull x-ray from the
side

SPECIALISED X-RAYS

Computerised axial tomography (CAT) scan

The CAT scanner is an x-ray device for obtaining pictures of the brain with no discomfort to the patient. The x-rays pass through the patient's head to a detector connected to a computer. The x-ray source and the detector rotate around the patient's head, taking readings from many angles. The computer translates the readings into television pictures, which appear as thin slices of the patient's head. Sometimes an injection of an iodine compound is given into a vein in the patient's arm to show even more detail of the brain.

There are innumerable indications in neurological practice for a CAT scan, which because of its very great sensitivity is able to detect very small abnormalities. Such indications range from suspected tumours (see Chapter 12), congenital structural abnormalities (see Chapter 4), hydrocephalus (see Chapter 4), abnormalities of blood vessels (see Chapter 5), brain abscesses (see Chapter 10), collections of blood following trauma (see Chapter 11) and sometimes in the presence of suspected degenerative disorders of the brain (see Chapter 8).

The child having a CAT scan has to lie very still for about 15 minutes while the top of the head is within the scanner machine (Fig. 3/3). Because of the need to be perfectly still for more than a few seconds, younger children will almost always require either heavy sedation or a short general anaesthetic. Figures 3/4, 3/5 and 3/6 show the normal and abnormal appearances from a CAT scan.

Angiography

This is a technique in which a radio-opaque dye is injected into an artery. In neurological practice angiography has been used extensively to define abnormalities within the brain due either to

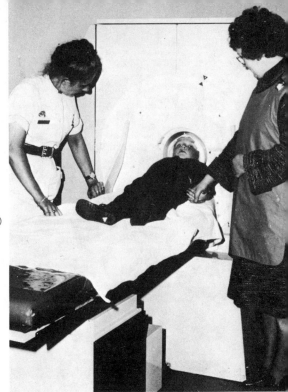

Fig. 3/3
Computerised axial
tomography (CAT scan)

tumours which will distort the normal course of the brain
blood vessels or abnormalities of the vessels themselves, such as
aneurysms or congenital abnormalities of the vessels (Figs. 3/7a
and b; 3/8). This technique is less frequently used than previously
due to the advent of the CAT scan.

The dye is either injected into the carotid or vertebral arteries in
the neck or through a long catheter threaded through a large bore
needle placed in the femoral artery in the groin. A general
anaesthetic is usually required for children although it is feasible
to perform angiography using only a local anaesthetic at the site of
the injection.

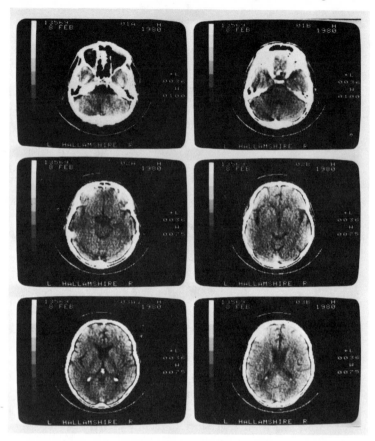

Fig. 3/4 A normal adult CAT scan. The black area is the CSF in the ventricles
of the brain, and the three white areas in the bottom left hand picture are
calcium in the choroid plexi of the lateral ventricles (see Chapter 4). The views are
as if one is looking down onto the head with the eyes towards the top of each
picture. Reading from left to right and down the six pictures, the 'slices' are
getting gradually higher up the brain

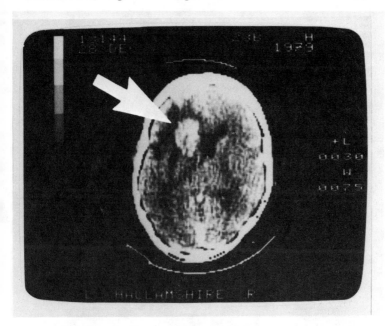

Fig. 3/5 A large tumour demonstrated on a CAT scan

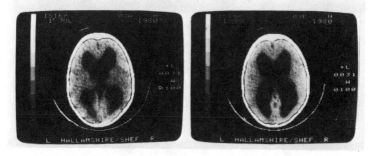

Fig. 3/6 Large ventricles due to hydrocephalus demonstrated on a CAT scan

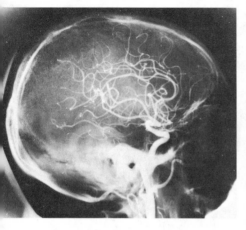

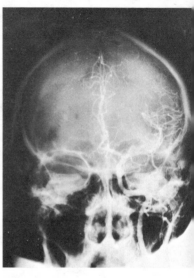

Fig. 3/7a (*above*) Carotid angiogram (side view)

Fig. 3/7b (*right*) Carotid angiogram (front view)

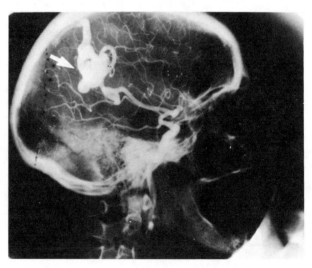

Fig. 3/8 Carotid angiogram demonstrating a large arterio-venous malformation (see Chapter 5)

Myelography

This is an examination of the spinal cord. The principle is to introduce a dye into the subdural space around the cord that therefore demonstrates its shape and also its movement within the spinal column. A radio-opaque dye may be used or air may be injected. The injection is usually performed by means of a lumbar puncture (see below). Following the injection the dye or air is allowed to run up the spinal column around the cord by tilting the patient head down, and down the canal and around the cord and cauda equina (the sheath of nerves that are the continuation of the spinal cord and the nerves for the lower part of the body) by tilting the patient head up (Fig. 3/9).

The indications for myelography include, a suspected tumour or other pressure (as from a disc) on the spinal cord which will interrupt the flow of the dye or contrast past the point of the pressure (myelographic block), a tumour of the spinal cord itself, or one of the structural abnormalities that may interfere with the function of the cord (see Chapter 4) (Figs. 3/10 and 3/11).

Myelography in children is nearly always undertaken with a general anaesthetic. A stay in hospital after the examination for 24 hours is advisable due to the relatively frequent occurrence of headaches—sometimes quite severe.

A variety of other specialised x-ray investigations are available to evaluate any patient with suspected neurological disorder. Major advances continue to be made in refining these investigations.

ELECTROPHYSIOLOGICAL INVESTIGATIONS

Electroencephalography (EEG)

Electroencephalography is the measurement of the electrical waves from the brain. We all have electrical brain waves and if we are able to amplify these through a series of electronic amplifiers,

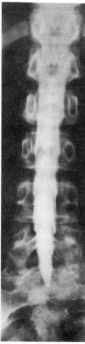

Fig. 3/9 (*left*) A normal myelogram (radio-opaque dye)

Fig. 3/10 (*below left*) Myelogram demonstrating a block (myelographic block) due to the pressure of a small tumour on the cord

Fig. 3/11 (*below right*) Myelogram demonstrating a distortion of the lower end of the spinal cord due to bony abnormality of the spinal column which fixes the cord and splits it into two (see diastometamyelia, Chapter 4)

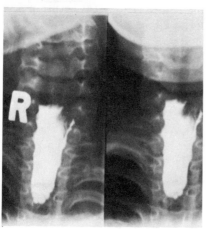

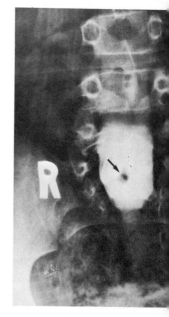

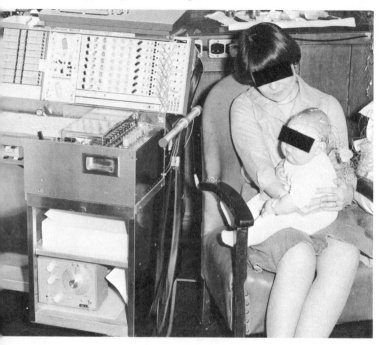

Fig. 3/12 Recording an electro-encephalograph (EEG)

then it is possible for these to be recorded onto a paper. This is essentially the technique of electroencephalography. Recordings are made by fixing electrodes to the head or skull (Fig. 3/12). Needles are not used as electrodes.

Nowadays the EEG is most often employed to evaluate possible epilepsy (Chapter 17). Although the diagnosis of epilepsy depends principally upon description of the attacks in question, the EEG is particularly useful in categorising the more specific nature of the attacks and may be helpful in the management of the more difficult epilepsies. In epilepsy the normal brain wave pattern may be altered (Figs. 3/13 and 3/14).

For the child the only fear of an EEG will be that of the

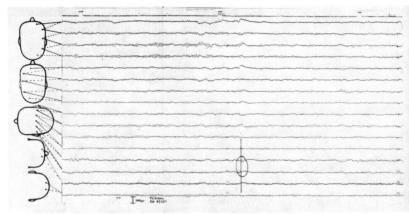

Fig. 3/13 A normal EEG tracing

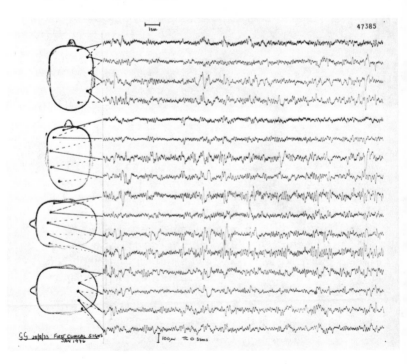

Fig. 3/14 The EEG tracing of a patient with epilepsy

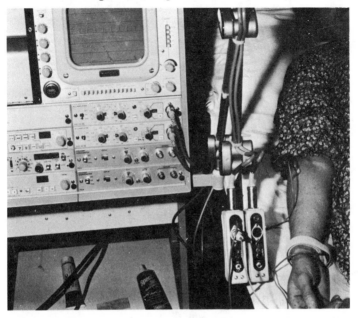

Fig. 3/15 An electromyographic (EMG examination)

unknown. The electrodes used are only attached to the skull by special electrode jelly and the whole recording lasts usually no more than 20 minutes.

Electromyography (EMG)

It is possible, as with EEG, to record electrical activity from active muscle fibres. The function of nerves may be studied by stimulating with electrical impulses at different points in their course and thereby estimating the speed at which the impulses are conducted. With a small needle (acting as an electrode) inserted into a muscle it is possible to study the electrical activity of the muscle directly (Figs. 3/15 and 3/16). The normal electrical activity of muscle is known and the alterations that occur if there is disease of

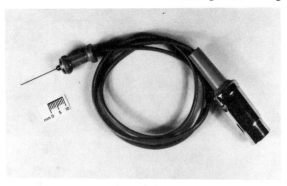

Fig. 3/16 An EMG needle electrode

either the nervous control of muscle activity or of the muscle itself is also known.

For the child undergoing electromyographic examination this is usually split into two parts. The first part of the examination is the study of nerve function by electrical stimulation. Following this the direct examination of muscle activity is made by the insertion of a needle electrode into muscle. Most children tolerate the electrical stimulation of a nerve being rather like the sensation of 'banging the funny bone', but naturally are less tolerant of the needle electrode studies. However, as such, the needle is not particularly painful although the prospect of the needle is something that upsets children—and adults.

LUMBAR PUNCTURE

The examination of the cerebrospinal fluid (CSF) has always been an important neurological examination, although in recent years its value has been restricted predominantly towards the diagnosis of infections of the CSF as in meningitis (see Chapter 10), and in a small number of other neurological conditions in which alterations in the protein content of the CSF may be diagnostically useful.

The usual procedure for lumbar puncture is that the patient lies on the side, usually the left, with the head bent forward and the knees flexed up towards the body (Fig. 3/17).

A lumbar puncture needle contains within it a solid trochar and is inserted through the gaps in the vertebral bodies of the spine at the level of the top of the hip bones. The needle is directed through the thick dural layer of the spinal cord. When this is achieved the trochar is removed and CSF flows through the needle and may be collected and samples taken to a laboratory. At the time of the lumbar puncture it is possible to measure the pressure of the CSF by attaching a manometer to the end of the needle. Lumbar puncture should never be undertaken if there is a

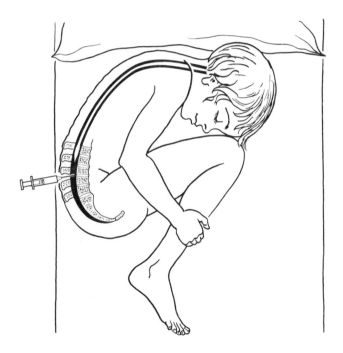

Fig. 3/17 Lumbar puncture: position of the patient

suspicion of raised intra-cranial pressure (Chapter 12) as this may be dangerous.

In the case of the very young (newborn) infant, lumbar puncture is undertaken with no preparation apart from that of the usual antiseptic procedures. In the older infant or young child some sedation or a light general anaesthetic is employed.

DEVELOPMENTAL ABNORMALITIES OF THE CENTRAL NERVOUS SYSTEM

4. The structurally abnormal nervous system

Children may be born with obvious structural abnormalities of the central nervous system. Such abnormalities may be gross and incompatible with normal life and survival, e.g. anencephaly (see below). Others may have more minor but obvious structural defects which need careful assessment and investigation to determine their significance, e.g. craniosynostosis (see below). Some structural abnormalities will not be obvious but may eventually produce neurological dysfunction, e.g. diastometamyelia (see p. 73). The careful examination of newborn infants is very important in the early detection of some of the less obvious abnormalities.

Major structural abnormalities of the brain and spinal cord are common and a large number of deaths in the first year of life are due to such abnormalities, as are a large number of intra-uterine deaths. A knowledge of central nervous system (CNS) embryology is necessary to understand completely the mechanism of such defects. The brain and spinal cord are formed by the 'folding' of nervous tissue—failure, or partial failure of this folding causes most of the structural abnormalities of the CNS.

ANENCEPHALY

The term anencephaly refers to the absence of a brain and is obvious at birth and can be diagnosed prenatally with a scan. The cause of the failure of the fusion of the neural tubes in early fetal life is unknown. However, there is a close association with spina bifida, and the defect occurs more often in the children of very young mothers. In the Western world it is the most common structural abnormality of the brain, occurring in approximately

1.18 per 1 000 births; it appears more often in some ethnic groups and may have a familial tendency.

The appearance at birth is characteristic. There is almost no cranium, although the face and eyes may be reasonably well developed. Anencephalic infants have a head and face that vaguely resemble those of a frog. The presence of anencephaly is suspected in utero with the finding of a high level of a protein known as alphafetoprotein (AFP) in the maternal blood and in the liquor amnii. This test is now used to screen for several of the central nervous system malformations in early fetal life. High levels in the blood are indicative of exposed fetal neural tissue and need to be confirmed by amniocentesis and an ultrasonic scan. An offer of termination of pregnancy could then be made. Hydramnios (an excess of liquor in the uterus) is common in pregnancies in which the fetus is anencephalic. This is probably due to impaired fetal swallowing.

After birth some automatic reflex activity may exist in these infants but there is no higher-brain activity. Survival is seldom for more than a few hours. The chances of recurrence in future pregnancies are high—as high as one in 20.

With an increase in AFP screening the incidence of anencephalic children being born should fall.

SPINA BIFIDA

This term simply refers to the failure of the bones of the spinal column to fuse in the midline. By itself it is of no real significance and spina bifida (occulta) of the lumbar vertebra 5 and sacral vertebra 1 is a common incidental finding on x-ray.

What is significant is spina bifida associated with a failure of development of the spinal cord and the spinal nerves.

Two groups of maldevelopment are recognised. In the first there is the myelomeningocoele, in which a large defect exists allowing the spinal cord and nerves to be exposed directly to the surface, with at the best only a thin membrane covering them (spina bifida cystica) (Fig. 4/1). In this condition, AFP levels in the maternal blood and amniotic fluid will be high. In the second

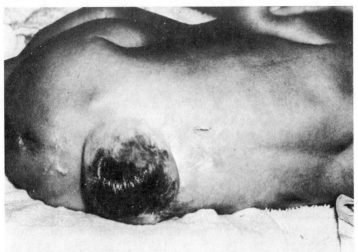

Fig. 4/1 Spina bifida cystica

group is the meningocoele, where there is a complete covering for the nervous tissue by skin and therefore there will be normal AFP levels. In both the abnormalities there will be a protrusion onto the surface in the midline. The more common of the two abnormalities is the myelomeningocoele. Both the defects are more common in the lumbar, lumbo-thoracic or lumbo-sacral areas. The incidence of the two abnormalities together is approximately 1.5 per 1 000 births with considerable regional variation throughout the United Kingdom.

The term spina bifida, then, is used to describe the two conditions—myelomeningocoele and meningocoele.

Hydrocephalus (see below) commonly develops in association with spina bifida defects of the type described above. This may be due to the spinal cord being tethered and thus causing traction on the brain in fetal life. This could then result in the brainstem and medulla being 'pulled down' through the opening in the base of the skull (foramen magnum), so interrupting the normal flow of cerebrospinal fluid (CSF).

The abnormality of the spinal nerves in the lumbar and sacral regions results in varying degrees of dysfunction of the bladder, bowels, and legs in children with either a myelomeningocoele or meningocoele.

With meningocoeles the abnormalities are usually minor but less so with myelomeningocoeles. Usually with the latter there is profound weakness with lack of sensation in the legs and paralysis of bladder and bowel. The degree of weakness and its distribution will vary with the level of the defect and with this the amount of damage to the nerves and spinal cord. A varying neurological picture may emerge: there may be complete loss of function below a certain level; paralysis over several nerve segments but with some activity distally from isolated cord activity; a combination of spasticity with a little voluntary activity; or occasionally paralysis of one leg with the other remaining almost unaffected. Abnormal postures and deformities of the feet are common and partly determined by which muscle groups are still active. Spinal deformity (kyphosis) is often seen.

If there is only minimal leg involvement bladder function may be normal or near normal. If there is no activity below the muscle groups innervated by the sacral nerves then it is unlikely that the bladder will be able to empty in the usual way and bladder sensation will be impaired. Manual bladder pressure is required in such children to achieve complete urinary voiding.

Management

Of immediate concern is the surgical repair of the defect in the back in those children where there is no skin covering. This prevents infection and further damage to the exposed nervous tissue. Surgery is usually carried out within the first few days of life.

The next problem that commonly has to be tackled in such a child is the treatment of hydrocephalus, which may be apparent at birth or in the first few weeks of life (see p. 66).

A careful evaluation of bladder and kidney function is necessary because bladder paralysis can have profound effects on the whole of the genito-urinary system. Urinary infections are common.

After the newborn period, particular attention is given to making the best use of the muscle power that exists in the legs and the feet. Orthopaedic intervention is required. Extensive lower limb splintage is necessary for ambulation. Despite such surgical activities, often over several years, relatively few children with myelomeningocoele walk, even with splintage.

The long-term management of urinary incontinence requires, in the male, the wearing of a penile appliance. In the female it has been common for the ureters to be transplanted into a loop of the small bowel which is brought to the surface of the abdomen (ileal conduit). More recently, management has been with either an indwelling urinary catheter or intermittent self-catheterisation.

Attention to the bowels is important because of the impaired innervation of the rectum. Complete constipation or, alternatively, faecal soiling needs to be avoided by active bowel management.

In summary, spina bifida, or the combination of spina bifida and hydrocephalus, poses a lifetime of treatment of the numerous problems that are experienced by such children. Despite extensive treatment these individuals remain very handicapped. Experience has questioned the wisdom of treating all those with spina bifida. In the severely affected it has been suggested that only nursing care should be given at the time of birth, since mortality will be 100 per cent. Notwithstanding the purely medical aspects of spina bifida, young persons, some of whom are mentally retarded (because of hydrocephalus), can have emotional difficulties with low self-esteem and sexual impotence, giving very poor prospects for employment and even less for marriage.

Although the occurrence of spina bifida is not genetically determined in Mendelian terms it is more common in some geographical areas, and once a child has been born with the condition the chances of another similar offspring being born to the parents increases from 1.5 per 1 000 births in the United Kingdom as a whole to one in 20.

ENCEPHALOCOELE (CRANIUM BIFIDUM)

The meningocoeles and myelomeningocoeles described above occur in the lower part of the central nervous system. Similar defects can occur at the cranial end of the CNS; most commonly in the back of the head through a bony defect. The incidence is about one in 10 000 births. Rarely, such a defect occurs in the roof of the nose or the orbit of the eyes. These swellings are known as encephalocoeles and the sac that usually appears at the back of the head may or may not contain nervous tissue.

If an adequate skin covering exists, early surgery is not indicated. If this is not the case it is necessary to prevent possible rupture. The outlook depends on whether the sac contains nervous tissue. There may be difficulty in replacing the brain inside the cranium and some excision of brain tissue may be necessary. If so, blindness, epilepsy and mental retardation are common in survivors.

The subsequent development of hydrocephalus is common whether or not there is brain tissue within the sac.

HYDROCEPHALUS

Hydrocephalus implies that there is an excessive amount of CSF within and around the brain. There are several reasons for this and before they can be considered in detail it is necessary to understand the manufacture and circulation of CSF.

Cerebrospinal fluid is formed by the secretory and filtering activity of the ependymal lining of the choroid plexi in the lateral, third, and fourth ventricles (or cavities) of the brain. The fluid circulates through the ventricular system of the brain and the subarachnoid space that envelops both the brain and the spinal cord (see Chapter 2).

Most of the CSF is formed in the two lateral ventricles which connect with the slit-like third ventricle via the foramen of Monro. The third ventricle connects by the narrow cerebral aqueduct within the mid-brain to reach the diamond-shaped fourth ventricle. The roof of the fourth ventricle is formed by the cerebellum. The CSF will pass from here through three apertures. One, known as the foramen of Magendie, is in the midline and two are at the sides of the ventricle—the foramina of Lushka. From the ventricular system the CSF passes over the surface of the brain and spinal cord beneath the arachnoid layers (within the subarachnoid space). Reabsorption is through the dural venous sinuses into which project arachnoid granulations.

Cerebrospinal fluid affords a protective jacket to the brain and is partially responsible for the intracranial pressure.

The amount of CSF may be increased because of a failure of reabsorption, and obstruction to its flow within the brain; when there is a loss of brain substance, with a compensatory increase in CSF; and rarely when there is an increased production due to a tumour of the choroid plexus.

With the failure of reabsorption, obstruction to flow, or over-production of CSF, signs of raised intracranial pressure may develop (see Chapter 12).

Hydrocephalus may be considered in two major groups: non-communicating and communicating. In the former the block to flow is within the ventricular system of the brain, whereas in the latter the circulation is obstructed somewhere between the exit from the brain itself and the arachnoid granulations that project into the venous sinus—a block to reabsorption. Division into these two groups can never be exact. Obstruction to flow can occur both within the ventricular system and outside it in the same patient. What is more important is the cause of obstructed flow.

NON-COMMUNICATING HYDROCEPHALUS

The common association of hydrocephalus with meningocoeles, myelomeningocoeles, and encephalocoeles is because of the likely presence of the so-called Arnold Chiari malformation. This malformation can be classified as Type I, II or III, depending partly on severity. In all three there is some degree of kinking of the medulla of the brain with protrusion of parts of the cerebellum through the foramen magnum. Obstruction may therefore occur to the flow of CSF out of the fourth ventricle.

Type I Arnold Chiari malformation seldom creates clinical problems before late childhood or adult life. The problems that may occur are due to the development of raised intracranial pressure (see Chapter 12) and the symptoms may include headache, neck pain, paralysis of the lower cranial nerves resulting in dysfunction of the palate and tongue, and also unsteadiness (or ataxia).

Type II Arnold Chiari malformation is the commonest and is particularly associated with meningocoeles and myelomeningocoeles.

Type III Arnold Chiari malformation includes not only the protrusion of median aspects of the cerebellum through the foramen magnum but a cervical spina bifida through which there will be herniation of brain tissue. This is most usually recognised as an encephalocoele.

Stenosis of the narrow aqueduct within the mid-brain may occur at the same time as an Arnold Chiari malformation, but more commonly it occurs alone. It may occur from a possible structural abnormality of the brain, secondary to the presence of a nearby tumour, a major abnormality producing distortion of the brain substance, or scarring from inflammation or infection in fetal or postnatal life.

COMMUNICATING HYDROCEPHALUS

An impairment to the complete circulation and therefore of the reabsorption of CSF may result from previous infection and inflammation of the meningeal coverings around the brain. Well-known examples of this are tuberculous and other meningitic infection, and haemorrhage either at birth or later. Such inflammations or infections can also quite easily be responsible for an obstructive or non-communicating hydrocephalus by interrupting the ventricular system itself.

Treatment and management

The head size may already be increased at birth in the infant with spina bifida because of the high intracranial pressure. An increase in the rate of growth of the head is usually seen in the first few days or weeks of life. The fontanelle (or soft spot) may be full, the eyes may have a downward look (sun-setting phenomena) and tapping of the skull may give a hollow-sounding note. A brain scan will show a marked increase in the size of the ventricles of the brain with a compression and thinning of the brain tissue. Similar signs will be seen in the other forms of hydrocephalus that are not due to an Arnold Chiari malformation. In the older child whose skull sutures have fused, the signs will be those of raised intracranial pressure (see Chapter 12, p. 155).

Attempts have been made to treat hydrocephalus by conservative means such as bandaging of the head and giving certain drugs. In most cases some surgical operation is required, using one of the many forms of silastic catheters fed into the lateral ventricles of the brain through a hole made in the skull (a burr hole). This catheter is connected to a one-way valve system (the shunt system) which is usually placed behind the ear and underneath the skin and connects to another catheter which passes (internally) down the neck to end either in a large vein in the heart (a ventricular-atrial shunt), the pleural cavity of the chest (a ventricular-pleural shunt), or the peritoneal cavity of the abdomen (a ventricular-peritoneal shunt) (Fig. 4/2). The valve within the system (and there are many different types of valves) ensures not only that the flow of CSF is in one direction but also (by having a suitable opening pressure) that the brain's ventricular pressure is maintained at about normal.

Unfortunately, shunt systems may be associated with problems. If the pressure in the ventricles is allowed to drop too quickly when a shunt is inserted, haemorrhage from the vessels surrounding the brain may occur, or the skull bones may 'collapse

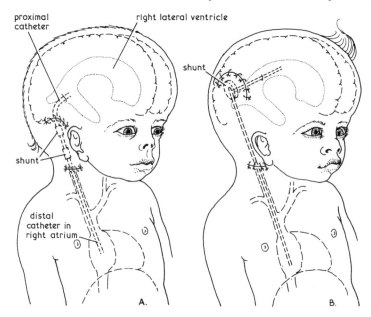

Fig. 4/2 Shunt systems for the treatment of hydrocephalus. A. Spitz-Holter; B. Pudenz

down' causing premature fusion. A sudden release of pressure may cause the brain to move upwards: upward coning. Complications are usually avoided if a medium pressure valve is inserted and slow initial drainage ensured. Shunt system blockages occur most commonly at the top or lower end and may require re-operation. The signs of this blockage may simply be raised intra-cranial pressure; often the early signs may be non-specific. A fall off in intellectual function, visual disturbance, a squint, or prominence of the veins on the forehead may suggest that the child has raised intracranial pressure. Parents or school teachers may be the first to recognise these diagnostic clues.

Infection of the shunt system can occur, leading to septic emboli circulating in the blood and subsequent secondary infective problems such as sub-acute bacterial endocarditis. There is also an association between the development of nephritis and the presence of a shunt. There is very often a need to revise shunts, partly owing to the growth of the child—although elective revision at intervals is less advocated than before and surgical intervention advocated only when problems occur.

Children with hydrocephalus have variable mental ability. Many are severely retarded, others exhibit the so-called 'cocktail party' personality in which superficially they appear to be intellectually bright but such an appearance is illusory, and some are of normal or near normal intelligence.

Epilepsy is common, particularly in those that have troublesome shunts or have developed hydrocephalus secondary to an infection.

STRUCTURAL ABNORMALITIES ASSOCIATED WITH A LARGE HEAD

There are various structural abnormalities in which infants have large heads and these have to be distinguished from hydrocephalus. Careful clinical and radiological evaluation is vital to achieve an accurate diagnosis, at least, for prognostic and genetic advice.

A large head (macrocephaly) may be due to increased brain tissue (megencephaly) and megencephaly occurs with some storage disorders (Tay-Sachs disease, Hurler's disease; see Chapter 8) and other degenerative disorders of the brain (e.g. Alexander's disease).

Radiological evaluation and, in many cases, pathological studies of infants with large heads will reveal various rare structural abnormalities. Examples include holoprosencephaly (failure of the two cerebral hemispheres to form—often associated with abnormalities of midline facial development); agenesis of the corpus callosum (this may be a partial or total failure of development of the broad band of connective tissue between the two cerebral hemispheres); lissencephaly (a failure of the sulci (grooves) in the cerebral hemispheres to form); the Dandy-

Walker malformation (a developmental anomaly of the fourth ventricle resulting in a cystic dilatation of the ventricle, hydrocephalus, and underdevelopment of the surrounding brain tissues); and hydrancephaly (most of the cerebral hemispheres being absent owing to either a destruction or a developmental anomaly early in fetal life—a light shone through the head will demonstrate a virtual absence of brain tissue).

MICROCEPHALY

A small head usually suggests a small brain and most children with microcephaly have lowered intelligence. Microcephaly can be split into primary and secondary forms.

PRIMARY MICROCEPHALY

This is when the small size of the head is very apparent at birth—transmitted as an autosomal recessive condition. It may also be associated with a number of chromosomal abnormalities and non-chromosomal conditions such as Rubinstein-Taybi syndrome, Smith-Lemli Opitz syndrome or the Cornelia-de-Lange syndrome (see Chapter 16). In Aicardi's syndrome, which is X linked and lethal in males, the principal features in a female heterozygote infant are primary microcephaly, infantile spasms associated with the maldevelopment of the corpus callosum, and punched-out lesions in the retina of the eyes.

SECONDARY MICROCEPHALY

This can arise from various factors such as infection, anoxia, and traumatic delivery, in the last part of pregnancy or in the perinatal period. Irradiation of, and some biochemical disorders in, the mother may also be causative. In these conditions the head tends to grow very slowly, although initially of normal size.

Careful evaluation of such children is important for prognostic and genetic reasons. As well as the common association with mental retardation a microcephalic child may have epilepsy, behavioural difficulties, and cerebral palsy.

CRANIOSYNOSTOSIS

At birth the bones of the skull are not formed together but connected only through their sutures. This is essential so that moulding of the skull may take place during childbirth and the brain may subsequently grow normally. Premature fusing of the skull bones will result in an abnormal development of the shape and the size of the skull and brain.

A wide variety of premature fusions of these bones exists. If the main suture which runs between the forehead and the back of the head (the sagittal suture) fuses early then the head will be long and thin (scaphocephaly). If the major suture that is at right angles to the sagittal suture (the coronal suture) is prematurely fused then a shortened head (brachycephaly) will result. Numerous other varieties occur, including a rare situation in which all the sutures are fused together prematurely. The differentiation of total craniosynostosis from microcephaly is important.

In many of the varieties of craniosynostosis early surgery will prevent the development of an abnormally shaped head or increased intracranial pressure. Surgical techniques have been developed in which prematurely fused sutures may be separated. Surgery must be undertaken early in infancy in most cases if the best results are to be obtained. Particular hazards that may exist are raised intracranial pressure and abnormal pressure on the nerve to the eyes and to the eyes themselves, in addition to the effects of an unusually shaped head.

Craniosynostosis is a particular feature of Apert's syndrome (see Chapter 16) and is also part of a dominantly inherited condition known as Crouzon's disease.

SPINAL DYSRAPHIC DISORDERS

The meningocoeles and myelomeningocoeles described are examples of spinal dysraphic lesions. The term is, however, most often applied to a small but important group of malformations of the lumbo-sacral spine. These produce defects by the distortion and tethering of the lower spinal cord and the leash of nerves known as the cauda equina. The tethering and distortion of the cord increases as the spinal column grows, resulting in weakness and sensory impairment in the legs, and possibly leading to impairment of bladder control and inequality in the size of the legs and feet. The presence of a structural abnormality may be suspected by noticing hairy patches, dimples, or soft-tissue swellings on the skin of the lower back.

If such a problem is suspected then early intervention is essential, aided by plain x-rays and x-rays using dyes injected into the spinal column (a myelogram, see Fig. 3/9, p. 52). If an abnormality is identified surgery is usually undertaken, in some a bony spur, which splits the cord, will be found in the spinal column (diastometamyelia, see Fig. 3/11, p. 52); in others there will be fatty masses or fibrous cords that will be interfering with the movement of the cord within the canal. Usually, surgery will be helpful in preventing further functional deterioration. On the other hand, it has to be recognised that neurological recovery following surgery is not to be expected: prevention of further deficits being the priority.

The wide variety of structural disorders of the central nervous system demands an early evaluation of the exact nature of the disorder to give appropriate specific therapy, to prognosticate, to counsel parents, and to ensure that the child receives the maximum and most appropriate medical and social care.

FURTHER READING

Brocklehurst, G., Sharrard, W. J. W., Forrest, D. and Stark, G. (1976). *Spina Bifida for the Clinician.* Spastics International Medical Publications. Clinics in Developmental Medicine No 57. William Heinemann Medical Books Limited, London.

Till, K. (1975). *Paediatric Neurosurgery for Paediatricians and Neurosurgeons.* Blackwell Scientific Publications Limited, Oxford.

5. Abnormalities of the blood vessels of the nervous system

Lesions are of two types, congenital structural abnormalities and those caused by thrombosis or embolism.

STRUCTURAL ABNORMALITIES

There are several congenital malformations which affect the cerebral blood vessels. The most common are angiomas, which consist of a tangle of vessels, and aneurysms, which are thin-walled swellings present on vessels. Many different clinical problems can result from these malformations and the possibility of their existence must be kept in mind during the examination and investigation of any child with a neurological problem. On the other hand, malformations of the cerebral vessels may be incidental findings at autopsy having caused no symptoms during life.

Angiomas

Careful examination of the tangle of vessels which make up an angioma shows that small arteries connect directly with small veins. The normal capillaries that exist between arteries and veins are absent. Angiomas may also be known as *arterio-venous malformations*. These may present clinically in several ways, although it is relatively rare for angiomas to produce symptoms in childhood. If of sufficient size they may give rise to the symptoms and signs of a space-occupying lesion—the mass effect. Presenting features can be epilepsy, headaches, or focal neurological dysfunction. Raised intracranial pressure may also be present. As a result of the lesion gradually increasing in size the development of symptoms and signs may be insidious. Blood flow through angiomas may be very great and result in other parts of the brain being relatively depleted and therefore underperfused; this may occasionally result in a degree of dementia. Occasionally a murmur may be heard through a stethoscope placed over the skull; this is caused by the high blood flow through the angioma and the absence of capillaries so that the arterial blood enters the veins at a higher pressure than usual.

The presenting signs and symptoms of an angioma may be those of an acute intracranial bleed. This may be as an acute catastrophic haemorrhage, a bleed into the space around the brain (subarachnoid haemorrhage) or into the brain substance (intra-cerebral bleed). In a child a subarachnoid haemorrhage accom-panied by seizures strongly suggests the presence of an angioma or arterio-venous malformation.

Spinal angiomas may produce symptoms because of either their increasing size or their rupture. In the former the clinical picture may be of back pain with progressive paraplegia. A lumbar punc-ture may reveal changes in the spinal fluid and myelography will often reveal the characteristic picture of an angioma. Techniques exist in which angiography may demonstrate the arteries serving the angioma (see Fig. 3/8, p. 50).

Aneurysms

The so-called 'berry aneurysm' that most commonly presents by bleeding in adults is almost certainly congenital and may occasionally bleed in childhood. It is thought to start as a defect in the middle layer of the artery wall. This results in either a small, thin-walled swelling on the artery which may enlarge with high blood pressure and/or atherosclerosis (hardening of the arteries) in later life. Aneurysms may occur in association with a congenital structural abnormality of the aorta known as coarctation, or with polycystic disease, which can affect a number of body organs such as the liver and kidneys.

The clinical presentation of an aneurysm might be due to the pressure that it causes, or its rupture producing a subarachnoid haemorrhage, an intracerebral bleed or both.

Venous malformations

These malformations are rare; the most well known being the aneurysm of the great vein of Galen situated deep inside the brain. Not only may this rupture with catastrophic effects but its increasing size causes pressure on surrounding brain tissue.

MANAGEMENT

In addition to the symptoms and signs discussed, repeated subarachnoid haemorrhages render the diagnosis of an angioma, an aneurysm, or other vascular malformation a near certainty. A lumbar puncture is necessary to diagnose such a bleed. A CAT scan may indicate the probable diagnosis, but an angiogram is needed to establish the diagnosis and to define the exact location of the malformation and the main vessels that supply it.

Intracranial angiomas are often complex in their structure and situated in areas of the brain that render surgical removal impossible. Their size may in some cases be reduced by ligating some of the main feeding vessels. The greater use of the operating microscope in neurosurgery has improved results in this field. The same remarks may be made about spinal angiomas. More recently, techniques have been developed in which small particles can be injected into the abnormal vessels to occlude them (embolisation). This is a new technique and requires great skill on the part of radiologists with experience in this type of treatment.

With ruptured berry aneurysms the scope of surgery is greater but will still depend upon the general state of the patient (whether in coma or not) and the site of the aneurysm. The principal aim of surgery will be to clip the neck of the aneurysm to prevent further bleeding. Here again the operating microscope has been a great advance. With some inaccessible lesions, tying off the carotid artery has been the treatment of choice—the opposite carotid artery then supplies the other side of the brain through the anatomical circle of Willis (an arterial circuit at the base of the brain) into which both carotids feed before supplying blood to the whole brain.

THROMBOSIS

Occlusion of vessels by thrombosis, although rare, does occur in children. There are several causes of such thrombotic lesions; the most common is that of an infection leading to an arteritis. Additionally, trauma to the arteries in the neck, cyanotic heart disease and its associated polycythaemia (thickening of the blood) or various infections, occasionally including those of the intra-cranial venous sinuses, can cause thrombosis. In a child with an infection usually only manifesting as a febrile illness, a hemiplegia may rapidly develop with complete or almost complete resolution over a period of days or weeks. In these children it is believed that an inflammation or arteritis has occurred. In others thickening (hyperplasia) of the muscle layers of the vessels may give rise not only to a single acute hemiplegia but also to recurrent hemi-plegias. In this group recurrent paralyses may be examples of moyamoya disease, in which recurrent occlusions of the major vessels occur; an angiogram will show a profusion of enlarged minor vessels, giving a typical hazy appearance. This phenomena is apparently more common in the Japanese; moyamoya is a Japanese word meaning 'puff of smoke'. Seizures sometimes occur with the onset of the hemiplegia.

CEREBRAL EMBOLI

There are several situations that can give rise to emboli or particles within the circulation which, depending on their origin, may then lodge in the cerebral arteries.

If a cerebral embolus is suspected by the onset of focal neurological signs the most important task is to identify the source. The range of possibilities include arterial emboli from the right side of the heart, infective emboli from a major vessel, infected emboli from sub-acute bacterial endocarditis, fat emboli after a major fracture, and air emboli after major vessel surgery or major vessel trauma. A cerebral abscess may develop from an infected embolus.

Many children who have a thrombotic or embolic lesion present with an acute hemiplegia. The clinical presentation of those with structural abnormalities may similarly be an acute hemiplegia. Clearly it is important to recognise the range of diagnostic possibilities in such situations and investigate accordingly. The use of the CAT scan now allows for early non-invasive investigation, although other definitive radiological studies may also be required. Lumbar puncture is also often indicated. Other possible causes of acute hemiplegia need to be considered, e.g. hemiplegic migraine (Chapter 18), a Todd's paralysis after a seizure (Chapter 17), a focal infection such as a cerebral abscess, a tumour, and occasionally an unusual encephalitis (see Chapter 10). Therefore, all children presenting with an acute hemiplegia need a thorough evaluation and investigation.

FURTHER READING

Isler, W. (1971). *Acute Hemiplegias and Hemisyndromes in Childhood*. Spastics International Medical Publications. Clinics in Developmental Medicine Nos 41/42. William Heinemann Medical Books Ltd, London.

6. Chromosome disorders

Some disorders are known to be associated with abnormal *genes* and varying patterns of inheritance. These patterns have been considered in Chapter 1. Genes consist of deoxyribonucleic acid (DNA) and are grouped together to form *chromosomes*. There are several disorders which are associated with demonstrable chromosome abnormalities. This chapter will describe the more important of these after an initial introduction to normal and abnormal human chromosomal patterns.

The physical and mental characteristics of an individual are largely dependent upon the genes they inherit from both their parents. The normal human has 23 pairs of chromosomes, each being made up of groups of genes, half derived from the male and half from the female parent. Twenty-two are known as *autosomes* and one pair *sex chromosomes*. In the female there are two X sex chromosomes and in the male an X and a Y.

Chromosomes exist in all body tissues and can be readily cultured from white blood cells or fibroblasts grown from tissue culture of skin biopsy samples. Special staining techniques enable the chromosomes to be examined under a microscope. The pairs of autosomes may be arranged in a series of 22, in order of decreasing size, and these together with the pair of sex chromosomes are known as the *karyotype* (Fig. 6/1). Each pair may be referred to by a specific number, or in groups which are lettered from A to G.

While it is possible to examine chromosomes under a light microscope it is not possible to examine genes. The presence or absence of a particular gene can only be inferred by the effects produced and the patterns of inheritance, and reference has already been made to the usual genetic patterns—*recessive, dominant*, and *X linked*.

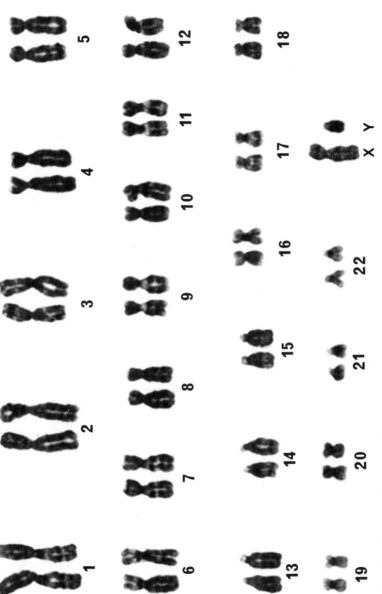

Fig. 6/1 The normal karyotype

Over the past 20 years several chromosomal disorders have been identified. These include in some conditions an extra chromosome, either an autosome or a sex chromosome, or the deletion (or absence) of a chromosome or part of it.

When the female egg is fertilised and the ovum is produced the 46 chromosomes from the female and the 46 from the male divide and then join together to form a *zygote* with 46 chromosomes—23 from each parent. This process does not always occur as perfectly as it should. Many such occurrences result in death of the zygote at this stage, but in some there can be survival with either an abnormal number of chromosomes or abnormal-size chromosomes. Some such children have recognisable groups of abnormalities. When an extra chromosome exists that is similar to a pair of autosomes the condition is called a *trisomy* and such a child has cells with 47 (not 46) chromosomes (Fig. 6/2). This is known as *non-disjunction*. Alternatively, during fertilisation autosomal pairs may become attached to form a compound chromosome or the compound chromosome may be inherited from one parent. This is known as *translocation* and the apparent total chromosome count will be 45 (Fig. 6/3). Seldom does any physical or intellectual abnormality result from this, perhaps because the total gene complement is normal. However, a translocation may be transmitted to offspring and result in physical and intellectual abnormalities because such children will have excess genes, although the total chromosome count in the offspring will be 46. A variety of further chromosomal abnormalities have been recognised more recently. These include *constrictions* in the body of the chromosome and *ring forms* in which the ends of a partially deleted chromosome become joined together.

One individual may occasionally have two distinct populations of chromosomes, some of which will be normal and some abnormal. This is known as *mosaicism*. Such individuals may be normal in all ways or have varying physical or intellectual abnormalities.

There are several syndromes in which abnormalities of chromosomes are particularly associated with mental handicap.

These can be abnormalities which affect the autosomes or abnormalities affecting the sex chromosomes.

DOWN'S SYNDROME (MONGOLISM)

Down's syndrome is the commonest specific syndrome associated with mental handicap and is due to a chromosomal abnormality. This disorder alone, with an incidence of one per 600 births in the United Kingdom, accounts for 30 per cent of children with known causes of severe mental retardation.

It occurs in all races and is more common in pregnancies where the mother is aged over 35. It has been known as a specific diagnostic entity since the last century but not recognised as a chromosomal disorder until just over 20 years ago. Most children with Down's syndrome have an extra chromosome with the 21 pair—trisomy-21 (Fig. 6/2), sometimes known as group G trisomy (non-disjunction). The total chromosome count will therefore be 47. In a very small proportion of patients with Down's syndrome the total chromosome count will appear to be normal at 46. In these cases the extra chromosome has become attached to another chromosome to form a translocation. The resultant compound chromosome has the appearance of a single chromosome but is of increased size. In these situations either parent may be a carrier of the translocation and have a total apparent count of 45. However, such translocations may arise sporadically. These two major groups of Down's syndrome are clinically similar although it is only with the trisomy-21, non-disjunction, that there is a strong association with increasing maternal age.

Down's syndrome is practically always easily recognisable at birth for the appearances are characteristic: the eyes slope downwards and inwards (mongoloid slant), the upper lids may overlap the lower and thus fold inside (epicanthic folds) against the nose, the ears are small and rounded, the tongue is large, transversely furrowed and tends to protrude. The iris of the eye will often be seen to have white spots within it, which are known as

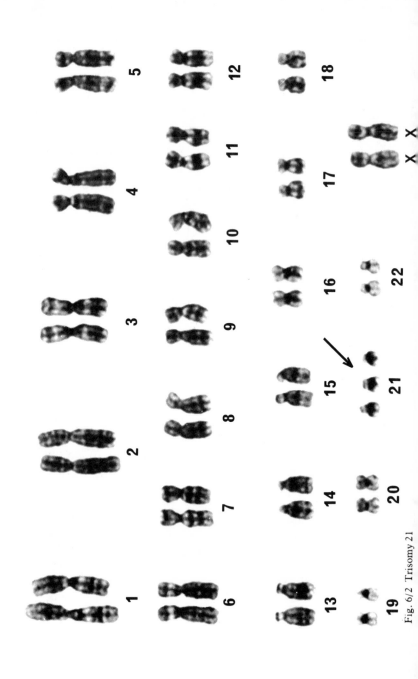

Fig. 6/2 Trisomy 21

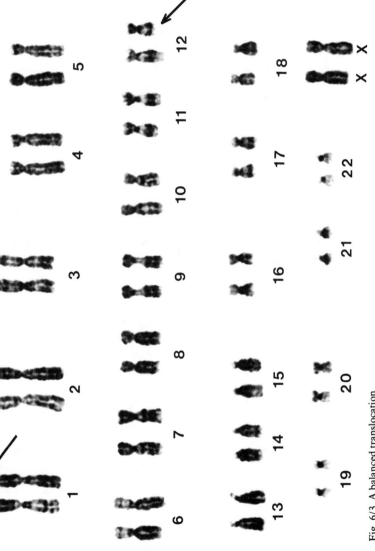

Fig. 6/3 A balanced translocation

Brushfield's spots. The neck and limbs are relatively short. The hands are short and stubby with often a single palmar crease (simian crease) rather than the more usual two, and the little finger may be short and incurving (clinodactyly). The large toe is widely separated from the next toe.

Babies with Down's syndrome are usually small and very floppy (hypotonic). Of the many features of Down's syndrome the most well known is the very high incidence of congenital heart defects of various sorts. Because of the severity of the heart defects in a number of children this association may contribute significantly to the mortality of those with Down's syndrome.

General development, both physical and mental, is slow. Physical size remains far below average. Mental development is slow, and this becomes more apparent with increasing age. While in all children with Down's syndrome there is mental retardation (when this is not the case the individual may be an example of a Down's mosaic) there is great variation between different individuals. The equable personality of patients with Down's syndrome is well known and their love for music, although not invariable, is often very striking.

A major hazard to health is the increased tendency that individuals with Down's syndrome have towards infections, particularly respiratory infections. This may be due to a general immunological impairment which is common and to the structure of the upper respiratory passages. Together with this there is a very high incidence of ear infections, serous otitis media, and deafness. The development of cataracts is also common.

Life expectancy is reduced, with many children dying before the age of five years. Despite this it is now realised that survival into and even past middle age is common—more common than previously thought and taught.

Diagnosis

Antenatal diagnosis is possible. A sample of fluid from around the fetus may be obtained by a needle inserted into the womb through the lower abdomen (amniocentesis). This is possible after 16 weeks of pregnancy. Cells from the amniotic fluid can be grown in a tissue culture and the chromosomal pattern examined. If examination reveals abnormalities associated with Down's syndrome termination of pregnancy may be offered. Because of the large increase in the incidence of Down's syndrome in women over the age of 35, these women should be offered amniocentesis. A mother who already has a child with Down's syndrome should also be offered amniocentesis, irrespective of her age.

The diagnosis at birth seldom presents any difficulty but should be confirmed by studying the karyotype from a sample of blood. This may identify the existence of a translocation, which is important for genetic counselling of the parents.

PATAU'S SYNDROME (TRISOMY-13-15)

This syndrome is characterised by severe mental retardation and other features, including a receding chin, a variety of eye defects, low-set ears, hare lip, cleft palate, and extra fingers and toes (polydactyly). It is far less common than Down's syndrome but is similarly related to increasing maternal age. Survival past six months is unusual.

Antenatal diagnosis is possible; however, the risk of recurrence is low unless one parent is a translocation carrier.

EDWARDS' SYNDROME (TRISOMY-17-18)

Several features overlap those in Patau's syndrome. Additionally, it is common to see antero-posterior elongation of the skull, webbing of the neck, congenital heart defects, overlapping fingers with an unusual position of the thumb, and so-called 'rocker bottom' feet.

Various abnormalities of skin creases are seen in Patau's and Edwards' syndrome and a study of these patterns (dermatoglyphics) may be diagnostically helpful.

Edwards' syndrome is also related to increasing maternal age but appears more common in girls. The risk of recurrence and the outlook for survival is similar to Patau's syndrome.

The three conditions just described are examples of chromosomal disorders in which the abnormality is associated with additional chromosomal material.

CRI-DU-CHAT SYNDROME

In the cri-du-chat syndrome there is a partial deletion of a short arm on chromosome number 5. The most specific clinical feature of this condition is the cat-like cry (cri-du-chat) that is present in infancy, although not later.

The syndrome, which appears to be more common in females, is also characterised variously by low birth-weight, slow growth, mental retardation, a small head (microcephaly), widely set eyes (hyperteleorism), epicanthic folds, downward slanting of the eyes (anti-mongoloid slant), and simian palmar creases. Apart from a simian crease, which is common in a number of chromosomal disorders, other dermatoglyphic abnormalities may often be seen in this syndrome.

Most commonly the syndrome arises sporadically, although occasionally one or other parent may be a translocation carrier.

SEX CHROMOSOME DISORDERS

There are several abnormalities of the sex chromosomes which are associated with recognisable syndromes.

In general the presence of an extra X chromosome tends to be associated with mental subnormality. In males the greater the number of X chromosomes the greater may be the degree of mental retardation and physical disorder. This is less so in females. The absence of an autosome appears to be a lethal condition, but not so the absence of a sex chromosome. We thus may have a syndrome in which the sex chromosome complement may be XO, as in Turner's syndrome (see below). In a normal female there are two X chromosomes and appropriate staining of body cells will demonstrate the presence of small masses known as Barr bodies. These small masses are sex chromatin, which exists beneath the membrane of the nucleus of any body cell which has two X chromosomes. This is not seen in the usual male karyotype, when there is only one X chromosome present. A normal female is therefore *chromatin positive*, whereas the male is *chromatin negative*.

KLINEFELTER'S SYNDROME (XXY)

This is the most common sex chromosome abnormality, occurring about once in every 500 males. There is a strong link with mental retardation, although not of a severe degree. With two X chromosomes present the individuals may be chromatin positive even though male.

Boys with Klinefelter's syndrome, although of near normal height in childhood, do not develop secondary sexual characteristics at puberty and there is a tendency towards a tall, thin stature with long limbs. Breast development (gynaecomastia) occurs in some and in later adult life, unless testosterone therapy is given, the body proportions tend towards obesity.

If the condition is suspected in childhood, when the clinical features may not be that obvious, the X chromatin material may be detected. This is done by scraping the inside of the mouth with a spatula (a buccal smear), providing cells which can be stained to look for the Barr bodies. This is a useful preliminary test.

TURNER'S SYNDROME (XO)

Ten per cent of children with Turner's syndrome are mentally retarded. As there is only one X chromosome present these individuals are chromatin negative. The principal clinical features are short stature with a female shape, a broad chest with unusually widely spaced nipples, swelling of the feet (oedema) in infancy, often webs on each side of the neck with a low hair line, an unusual angle at the elbow (cubitus valgus), a high incidence of heart abnormalities, particularly at the beginning of the aorta (coarctation of the aorta), and maldevelopment and malfunction of the ovaries. All these features are not necessarily found in every individual with Turner's syndrome, particularly if not all the cell population have the Turner's karyotype—Turner mosaicism.

As indicated, many of these conditions should be recognisable at birth. There is a need for early counselling of the parents as most of these children will need continuous care and special help. The need for careful genetic counselling should be obvious.

FURTHER READING

Emery, A. E. H. (1979). *Elements of Medical Genetics*, 5th edition. Churchill Livingstone, Edinburgh.

Kirman, B. and Bicknell, J. (1975). *Mental Handicap*. Churchill Livingstone, Edinburgh.

Siggers, D. C. (1978). *Prenatal Diagnosis of Genetic Disease*. Blackwell Scientific Publications Limited, Oxford.

Smith, D. W. (1976). *Recognisable Patterns of Human Malformation*, 2nd edition. Vol 7 in the series *Major Problems in Clinical Pediatrics* (Schaffer, A. J. (Ed)). W. B. Saunders Co, Philadelphia.

7. Cerebral palsy: the 'spastics'

Some children, as a result of brain damage acquired in fetal or early postnatal life, have a motor or physical defect known as cerebral palsy. This is a complex entity and has been difficult to define adequately. One accepted definition is of a motor disorder which is a manifestation of non-progressive brain damage sustained in early life. Expressed differently, it is a motor disorder consequent upon early brain damage recognised primarily by disordered movement and posture. It is important to recognise that although the original brain damage is accepted as non-progressive, the clinical picture will usually be modified with age.

The United Kingdom incidence of cerebral palsy is approximately two per 1 000 live births, although recent Swedish figures show a drop in this incidence. There is evidence that a similar fall is occurring in the United Kingdom and this has been attributed partly to improved obstetric and perinatal care.

The cause of cerebral palsy is thought to be multifactorial and associations with many events have been demonstrated. The most important of these are intra-uterine infections in early pregnancy, threatened abortions, generalised maternal illness, an episode in the third trimester of pregnancy such as toxaemia, antepartum haemorrhage, intra-uterine growth retardation, premature onset of labour, and difficulties during labour and delivery itself. Various events in postnatal life have also been shown statistically to be associated with the development of cerebral palsy; they include perinatal respiratory difficulties, hypoglycaemia, hypothermia, infection of the central nervous system, severe seizures in early infancy, high levels of bilirubin in the neonatal period, and brain injury. Many of these factors are common, especially those occurring in the antenatal period, but seldom cause any form of brain damage.

A detailed and careful record of the pregnancy, delivery and postnatal care of any child suspected of having cerebral palsy is essential. However, it is important not to attribute automatically the cause of a child's cerebral palsy to any one factor but to recognise that the aetiology in many is uncertain. In some forms there is a stronger aetiological association than in others, and in some cerebral palsy may be the result of a genetically determined malformation of the brain.

The clinical classification of cerebral palsy is based on the major patterns of motor dysfunction that are seen in individual children: hemiplegia, diplegia, quadriplegia, ataxia, hypotonia, dyskinetic and mixed types. Children with cerebral palsy are often known as 'spastics'. While such an interchange in terminology may be acceptable in a non-medical context, it is by no means appropriate in all children. Consideration of the major patterns alone is also not enough—patients with hemiplegia will very commonly have some abnormalities in the so-called unaffected side while those in whom the lower limbs are affected, as in diplegia, nearly always have some impairment of upper limb function. Indeed in any form of cerebral palsy the clinical picture may be a complex one, not only because the condition may change with time but also because the patient with a clinical picture dominated by spasticity (hypertonia) may have co-existent floppiness (hypotonia). The term spasticity alone is therefore limited, meaning no more than increased tone in the muscle when it is stretched, implying a defect in the control and regulation of voluntary movement. To use the name 'spastic' for these children is inaccurate.

Although recognising that considerable overlap occurs between the clinical forms of cerebral palsy described in this chapter there will be an individual description of the previously mentioned groups.

CLINICAL FORMS OF CEREBRAL PALSY

Hemiplegia

The large number of associated factors which may contribute to the development of cerebral palsy have been described above, although in at least a third of cases of hemiplegia it is difficult to identify reliably any possible cause. However, hemiplegic cerebral palsy has a particular association with cerebral vascular thrombosis either antenatally or perinatally, hypernatraemia, and occasionally encephalomyelitis. In those cases where no definite aetiology exists, an arterial embolus or thrombosis is believed to have occurred early in fetal life, the vessel in question having subsequently recanalised.

The arm is usually affected more than the leg and one of the earliest signs in hemiplegia may be abnormal fisting in the affected hand. In the first year there is commonly some increased stiffness in the affected arm with a reluctance to develop bimanual activity. The leg may be noted from an early age not to be kicked either in the same fashion or as much as in the non-affected leg and may be held straight and internally rotated. Onset of walking may be delayed but as long as there is no severe associated mental retardation this will eventually occur. When walking, the child with hemiplegia will be noted to have a tendency towards doing so on the toes of the affected side. Smallness of the affected arm and shortness of the leg are common, more so with increasing severity of the paresis.

Quadriparesis

This is sometimes referred to as 'double hemiplegia'. Most children so affected ultimately have very severe spasticity and the arms are more affected than the legs. While the term implies that all four limbs are affected this is seldom in a symmetrical fashion.

The aetiological factors that might be present in this variety of cerebral palsy are extensive and similar to those in hemiplegia.

Without doubt, this is one of the most severe forms of cerebral palsy and is often associated with profound mental retardation and marked feeding problems. Irritability in early infancy is very common.

Cerebral diplegia

This is one of the earliest forms of cerebral palsy described and is still sometimes referred to as Little's disease, after a description by Dr William Little in the middle of the last century.

This condition has a very strong association with prematurity and 'light-for-dates' infants. Postnatal causes of cerebral diplegia are rare. There has been a significant decrease in this form of cerebral palsy in recent years.

Most children with cerebral diplegia are initially hypotonic, although they may have a tendency towards so-called 'extensor thrusting'. If held upright there may be a tendency for the legs to be extended, adducted, and often to cross over due to increased tone in the adductor muscles of the thigh. This is referred to as 'scissoring'. The arms are usually held into the side, although very commonly in this form of cerebral palsy the upper limb function may be nearly normal. Sitting will be delayed and when it is achieved it will be in an unstable fashion, with the child sitting on the sacrum and leaning forward with a rounded back. This is due to spasticity and tightness of the hamstring muscles. Adductor spasm also causes a very small sitting base. Rolling over is difficult and there will be delay in starting to walk. When this does occur it will be with the knees and hips semi-flexed. The development of ankle, knee, and hip contractures is common.

Ataxic diplegia

The description above principally relates to the so-called spastic diplegia, but a diplegia with an added cerebellar impairment is also recognised. It has been suggested that this condition may be genetically determined in some children. Hypotonia is an early feature but improves slowly with age. There is a marked delay in motor development. When early grasping takes place there is a definite tremor, which should suggest cerebellar dysfunction. Spasticity is not as marked as in the more well-known diplegia. The gait will be broad based and stamping. Adductor spasm causing 'scissoring' is rare.

Ataxic cerebral palsy

Many authorities doubt the existence of this form of cerebral palsy as a separate entity, with good reason. Hypotonia and ataxia in a young infant may so often indicate some specific brain malformation or the early signs of a progressive illness, and such children need careful investigation and assessment.

The salient features ascribed to this condition include hypotonia with delayed motor milestones, a coarse tremor of the head, an intention tremor of the hands and truncal tremor on sitting and standing. There will be a broad-based gait.

Dyskinetic cerebral palsy

The characteristic feature of this form of cerebral palsy is irregular and involuntary movements of a number of muscle groups in the body. While some of these are present only on movement, some may be virtually continuous. The term *athetoid* is often used. This describes the typically slow and writhing movements, more commonly of distal muscles. In many children there are also quick and jerky movements, predominantly in the proximal muscles—so-called *chorea*. If both these types of movement disorder are seen together, the term *choreo-athetoid* is applied. In addition slow, often writhing movements may affect the muscles of the trunk and this is referred to as *dystonia*. These three disorders of muscle movement are often seen in the same child with dyskinetic cerebral palsy.

There is a strong, now almost historical, association with this form of cerebral palsy and kernicterus from hyperbilirubinaemia

caused by Rhesus disease. The highly successful prevention of
Rhesus disease by the administration of anti-D serum to Rhesus-
negative mothers who have evidence of antibody formation after
pregnancy has dramatically decreased the numbers of pregnancies affected by Rhesus incompatibility. Furthermore, the
organisation and centralisation of facilities for exchange transfusions in the few remaining affected infants has made this cause
of dyskinetic cerebral palsy rare. More commonly the cause is
severe damage to the nervous system, particularly from perinatal
hypoxia and congenital malformations.

Neurological abnormality is nearly always apparent in the
neonatal period. Generalised hypotonia with marked motor delay
is extremely common. Feeding difficulties are equally common
and persistent, exacerbated partly by involuntary movements of
the oral muscles. The so-called primitive reflexes are maintained
far beyond the normal age.

Voluntary movements of the limbs are slow to develop, very
poorly controlled, and often accompanied by a variety of involuntary movements. These latter problems become progressively
more marked and obvious in the second year of life. In most cases
of dyskinetic cerebral palsy there is an accompanying severe
spasticity, but the early hypotonia persists in a small number.
Intelligence may be normal in those with persistent hypotonia,
although communication difficulties do exist. Severe speech
difficulties are very common in all forms of dyskinetic cerebral
palsy.

Mixed cerebral palsy

How large this group becomes depends on how strictly other
forms of cerebral palsy are classified. Children diagnosed as
having a particular type of cerebral palsy may well have other
signs in addition to those that are expected. Examples of these are
the presence of abnormal signs in the upper limbs of a child with
cerebral diplegia, or the athetoid movements that may be seen in
the hands of a hemiplegic patient. The diagnosis of mixed

cerebral palsy is usually reserved for children who cannot be placed into another specific category.

PROBLEMS ASSOCIATED WITH CEREBRAL PALSY

A child with cerebral palsy rarely has only a motor disability. There are usually various other disabilities which need to be identified and catered for.

Vision and hearing

In children with cerebral palsy there is a high incidence of squints, severe refractive disorders and impaired visual acuity. Some with hemiplegia may additionally have defects of the visual fields.

There is a strong association between high-tone deafness and the dyskinetic form of cerebral palsy. Testing hearing in affected children may be difficult but it is vital.

Alterations in sensation and perception

Various sensory deficits may be identified in children with cerebral palsy, and these must be recognised for prognostic reasons. In hemiplegic cerebral palsy there may also be neglect of, and a general reluctance to use, the affected arm and hand.

Learning difficulties

These are common, particularly in language development. Possible reasons may include the relative physical and subsequent social isolation of such children. Severe learning problems may co-exist, even in the mild forms of cerebral palsy.

Intelligence

While most children with cerebral palsy are of lower than normal intelligence, it is important to recognise that a proportion will be intellectually normal. The complexity of many of the handicaps adds to the difficulties that low intelligence in its own right produces.

Epilepsy

Epilepsy is common with all forms of cerebral palsy, with an estimated prevalence of about 60 per cent. It is more common in hemiplegic cerebral palsy and can often be difficult to treat. The management of epilepsy is described in Chapter 17.

Emotional problems

If the emotional needs of children with cerebral palsy are not recognised and carefully managed to the same degree as the physical problems, then there is a real risk that the overall handicap may be increased.

Emotional disturbance and behavioural problems are common in children with severe cerebral palsy, and also occur in children who are mildly affected. This last group perhaps deserves special attention, as so often they will attend normal schools. As they grow older many will become increasingly aware that there are significant limitations on their activities on the sports field and in day-to-day activities in the classroom. This can lead to ridicule and social isolation by their peers and sometimes by their teachers, who do not understand the nature of their condition, especially if it is not easily recognised. Particularly vulnerable times may be at puberty, when the unusual walk of the hemiplegic child will contrast even more with that of his peers. This aspect of a child's life and development must be fully recognised.

MANAGEMENT AND TREATMENT

The complex nature of cerebral palsy makes it impossible to generalise about detailed management and treatment: the very extent and variability of the problems demand a team approach.

Although this is a non-progressive disorder, the signs and symptoms in individual cases can vary considerably with time. Such variation means that regular re-evaluation and re-assessment of a child with cerebral palsy is essential, not only by doctors but by all involved in the child's care.

The concept of a multidisciplinary approach in paediatric practice is now well accepted, but many forget that it originated chiefly in the field of cerebral palsy management. It is impossible for any one therapist alone to treat a child if she is not aware of the full extent of the child's ability and disability. This includes intellect, hearing, vision, and a knowledge of the medical problems that may co-exist.

With cerebral palsy there may be an abnormal period of retention of primary automatic reflexes and a delay in development of secondary automatic reflexes. Early diagnosis may be beneficial by enabling early stimulation with a variety of sensory inputs rather than the institution of stereotyped therapy.

Different forms of therapy have been developed over the years and of these many have become virtual household names with enthusiastic supporters. The very fact that there are such differing schools of thought must suggest that no single one has necessarily all the answers.

The therapist must surely be as important as the method of treatment, and it is beyond the scope of this book to discuss such methods. It is essential to make the one important general point—namely, that the relationship between the doctors, therapists, psychologist, teachers, nurses, the child, and the family is the most essential ingredient towards achieving good results.

The role of the therapist is not just to provide individual therapy but to bring the parents into the therapeutic arena and to teach them how they can first help their own child. It cannot be emphasised too strongly that with the overall management of cerebral palsy the parents must be regarded as essential therapists. Thus a partnership develops between the parents and the professionals.

Orthopaedic surveillance of these children is important. There is a high incidence of contractures, which may well respond to judicious orthopaedic surgery. Surgical release of shortened spastic muscles may also be beneficial. However, decisions about the nature of such operations and their timing require much care; here again the team approach is important.

Speech therapy, in its role towards coping with early feeding difficulties and in the stimulation and development of speech and language, is important to a large group of children with cerebral palsy. Advice on seating and daily living activities comes most usually from an occupational therapist, although in many cases a physiotherapist assumes this role.

The aim of treatment for any child with cerebral palsy is to enhance development and allow the attainment of an independent existence in society. This may not necessarily be a realistic goal with all children, but the aim must surely be to enable the individual child to relate as much as possible to the environment, with a hope that maximum independence of existence can result.

FURTHER READING

Bobath, B. and Bobath, K. (1975). *Motor Development in the Different Types of Cerebral Palsy*. William Heinemann Medical Books Ltd, London.

Drillien, C. M. and Drummond, M. B. (1978). *Neurodevelopmental Problems in Early Childhood: Assessment and Management* (Chapter 13). Blackwell Scientific Publications Limited, Oxford.

Finnie, N. R. (1974). *Handling the Young Cerebral Palsied Child at Home*, 2nd edition. William Heinemann Medical Books Ltd, London.

Levitt, S. (1977). *Treatment of Cerebral Palsy and Motor Delay*. Blackwell Scientific Publications Limited, Oxford.

DISORDERS AFFECTING CENTRAL NERVOUS SYSTEM FUNCTION

8. Deterioration in brain function—the neurodegenerative disorders

The maturation of the nervous system in infants and children is assessed by monitoring the speed and age of achieving certain developmental milestones (motor, social, and intellectual). With an impairment of maturation the attainment of milestones may be delayed or distorted. Such a delay may be accompanied by problems that in themselves point to neurological dysfunction such as epilepsy, spasticity or ataxia.

Central nervous system function is known to deteriorate in old age. This is demonstrated, for example, by decreased ability to remember facts, to see and to hear well. This may be acceptable in the elderly but is certainly not acceptable when it occurs in childhood.

Nevertheless, although individually rare, a large number of diseases do lead to degeneration of central nervous system function in childhood. This degeneration is recognised by a loss of previously attained milestones with, in some cases, the development of epilepsy and other neurological abnormalities.

Neurodegenerative disorders are those diseases which occur when the brain and possibly the peripheral nervous tissue undergoes structural and subsequent functional change. There are several causes for these diseases and they can be considered under the following headings:

1. Storage disorders
2. Sub-acute viral encephalopathy
3. Degenerative disorders (without identified storage of material).

The recognition of neurodegenerative disorders in childhood depends upon a clear history of a loss of previously achieved milestones. This has to be carefully distinguished from those children who have had consistently slow development from birth. There are situations which may mimic neurodegeneration. Unrecognised epilepsy, particularly of the minor motor variety, may impair both motor and intellectual function. Treatment of the epilepsy will improve such functional deterioration. In a few children with developmental delay secondary behavioural changes may occur, most commonly in the second or third year of life, and cause a loss of some skills.

STORAGE DISORDERS

This term, when applied to the central nervous system, implies the presence of an abnormal accumulation of a substance within the brain. There may also be an accumulation in peripheral nervous tissue as well as in other organs and tissues of the body.

In most of the disorders, the biochemical fault is at least partially understood and the absence or deficiency of certain enzymes has been recognised. Thus many of these disorders can now be regarded as types of *inborn errors of metabolism*. The abnormal material which accumulates may be a lipid (e.g. sulphatides, gangliosides or cerebrosides) or a compound sugar (e.g. mucopolysaccharide) and can be primarily within either the white matter or the grey matter of the brain. In the case of the former the early signs will be of motor dysfunction, and in the latter social and intellectual dysfunction with the frequent development of seizures.

Metachromatic leukodystrophy

This disorder is so named because the abnormal accumulation of sulphatides in the white matter of the brain and other tissues produces an unusual staining reaction with the dye Toluidine blue. The usual blue colouration seen with this dye is replaced by a greeny-brown colour—metachromasia. This accumulation of sulphatides with an accompanying low level of cerebrosides is due to low or absent activity of an enzyme called aryl sulphatase A, which is responsible for the conversion of the first compound into the second.

The clinical presentation is most commonly in the second year of life with either progressive paraparesis or ataxia. Progression is relentless and the affected child will soon be unable to walk if he has already learned to do so. The child will become quickly totally dependent, with progressive physical and later mental deterioration. Seizures are a late feature. In the early stages of this disease there may be clinical spasticity, sometimes with absent tendon reflexes. This unusual combination of signs is due to a concurrent peripheral neuropathy caused by the storage of the sulphatides within the myelin layer of the peripheral nerves. Death occurs six months to six years after presentation.

The diagnosis of this disorder is made by examining fresh specimens of urine in which cellular deposits will demonstrate intracellular metachromatic material after staining with Toluidine blue. This phenomenon is due to the storage of sulphatides in the kidneys, from which epithelial cells are shed into the urine. Neurophysiological examination will usually demonstrate a peripheral neuropathy. The definitive diagnosis is made by examining white blood cells in which the level of the enzyme aryl sulphatase A will be either diminished or frankly absent.

Metachromatic leukodystrophy is autosomally recessively inherited. Therefore, parents with an affected child have a one in four chance of having another child similarly affected. Prenatal diagnosis, although sometimes technically difficult, may be possible by examining the enzyme levels in fibroblasts from amniotic fluid.

Tay-Sachs disease (GM₂ gangliosidosis)

This disorder is still sometimes referred to as *amaurotic familial idiocy* because of the ultimate combination of blindness and dementia. A compound referred to as a GM_2 ganglioside is stored predominantly within the grey matter of the brain, as well as in some other tissues. Storage is thought to be caused by the deficiency of an enzyme called hexosaminidase A and occasionally also another enzyme called hexosaminidase B. There are several different clinical forms, of which the most common are the infantile or the late infantile forms.

INFANTILE FORM

The onset of the disorder is within the first six months of life and the first sign is often an excessive startle reaction to sound. A cherry-red spot at the macula of the optic fundus is seen due to the storage of the gangliosides within the fundus (Fig. 8/1). Later, optic atrophy leads to blindness. There is a loss of intellectual and motor milestones, together with dementia, inappropriate laughing (gelastic fits), and marked hypotonia progressing eventually to a spastic paraparesis. Seizures are common in the second year of life. A large head (macrocephaly) develops because of the excessive storage of the ganglioside within the brain tissue. Ter-

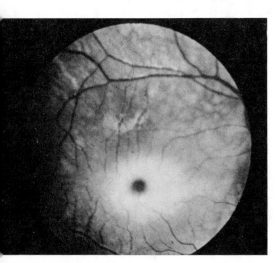

Fig. 8/1
The cherry red spot in
Tay-Sachs disease

minally there is decerebrate posturing with death most commonly by the age of four years.

LATE INFANTILE TAY-SACHS DISEASE (SANDHOFF'S VARIETY)

This has a later onset at between one and two years of age. Here again there is an excessive startle reaction to sound with progressive psychomotor deterioration and the early onset of fits. The so-called cherry-red spot is again seen at the macula of the optic fundus. As well as the cherry-red spot there may be a pigmentary retinitis and the development of blindness. Later a spastic paraparesis may occur. In this type of Tay-Sachs disease death occurs between the ages of four and ten years.

The diagnosis of Tay-Sachs disease is confirmed by estimating the levels of hexosaminidase enzymes in the blood. In an affected child they will be low or absent.

As with metachromatic leukodystrophy, Tay-Sachs disease is autosomally recessively inherited and it is also known to be more common in Ashkenazim Jews. Prenatal diagnosis from amniocentesis is feasible and technically often easier than with metachromatic leukodystrophy.

Mucopolysaccharidoses

There are several different forms of mucopolysaccharidosis. In all there is a defect in the metabolism of the complex sugars known as acid mucopolysaccharides (also known as acid glycosaminoglycans). The defect gives rise to a high urinary excretion of these compounds and their accumulation generally within the body.

Until comparatively recently seven varieties were described and often referred to as MPS I to MPS VII. More recently the further biochemical study of these disorders, the identification of relevant missing enzymes that are the explanation for the disordered biochemistry, and greater familiarity with the clinical forms suggest that at least 11 types of mucopolysaccharidoses exist.

MPS I (HURLER'S SYNDROME)

In this condition there is a high urinary excretion and body storage of two mucopolysaccharides—dermatan sulphate and heparan sulphate, due to the defect of an enzyme α-L-iduronidase.

These children are normal at birth and usually throughout the first year of life. In the second year development slows and a number of bony abnormalities develop because of the storage of mucopolysaccharides within the bone substance. X-rays will demonstrate thickening of the cortex of the humerus and, later, beaking of the lower thoracic vertebrae and widening of the ribs. The head will often be large and gross facial features gradually develop. The eyes are widely spaced, the nasal bridge is flat, the lips are large and the mouth is often open. There is often nasal obstruction and a high incidence of upper respiratory tract infections. A kyphosis develops at an early stage in this disorder. The hands are wide and the fingers short and stubby. The abdomen is protuberant, and there is often an umbilical hernia and marked enlargement of the liver and spleen (hepato-splenomegaly). The hair is coarse and profuse. Corneal opacities are common. All these features are thought to be due to the accumulation of the mucopolysaccharides in the tissues.

Eventually there is progressive spasticity, mental retardation, deafness, and optic atrophy. Death will occur in the first decade of life from bronchopneumonia or congestive cardiac failure since the lungs and the heart are also infiltrated with mucopolysaccharides. The condition is autosomally recessively inherited.

MPS II (HUNTER'S SYNDROME) (Fig. 8/2)

In this syndrome there is also a high body storage and urinary excretion of dermatan and heparan sulphate but this is caused by a defect of the enzyme iduronate sulphatase.

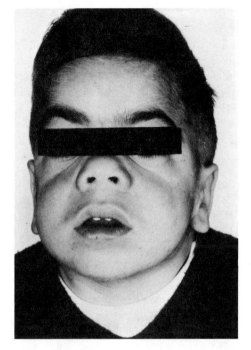

Fig. 8/2
Hunter's syndrome

In this form of mucopolysaccharidosis the clinical picture may be similar to Hurler's syndrome but less severe. It is an X-linked condition and occurs only in boys. Mental deterioration and corneal clouding are seen but are less obvious. Retinitis pigmentosa can lead to early complete blindness. There appear to be two clinical forms of Hunter's syndrome: a severe form with survival seldom past the teens and a mild form in which all the symptoms are less marked and survival can be into the fifth decade.

MPS III (SANFILIPPO'S SYNDROME TYPE A and B)

Heparan sulphate is the mucopolysaccharide that is excessively stored and excreted in the two forms of Sanfilippo's syndrome. The type A form is due to a defect of the enzyme heparan sulphate sulphamidase and the type B to a defect of α-N-acetyl-glucosaminidase.

Here there may be progressive intellectual deterioration starting in the third year of life with fewer physical signs than in the other forms of mucopolysaccharidoses described. Hepatosplenomegaly is less marked and the facial features are less coarse. The stature is short as in the other two forms and there may be well marked osteoporosis (thinning of the bone matrix), joint contractures, a short neck, prominent maxillae, and a short nose. There is occasional corneal clouding and survival may occur into young adulthood. This condition is autosomally recessively inherited.

IN SUMMARY

In investigating these conditions, urinary screening for the excessive amount of mucopolysaccharides is important not only in establishing a diagnosis but also in differentiating one form of mucopolysaccharidosis from another. In Hurler's, Hunter's, and Sanfilippo's forms of mucopolysaccharidoses, 20 to 40 per cent of the lymphocytes contain inclusions which stain metachromatically with Toluidine blue. X-rays of the long bones, skull, ribs, and vertebral bodies can be helpful diagnostic investigations.

Fibroblast culture allows the distinction of a male infant with Hunter's syndrome from one with Hurler's syndrome. In the two forms of Sanfilippo's syndrome fibroblast culture can differentiate type A from type B. Antenatal diagnosis using fibroblast cultures of the amniotic fluid is feasible in several of the mucopolysaccharidoses. The remainder of the mucopolysaccharidoses do not necessarily have any neurological features and in many the onset of symptoms and signs is in later life. Their names, classification, and biochemical features are summarised in Table 8/1.

	Syndrome	Enzyme defect	Major storage and urinary mucopoly-saccharide
I H I S I H-S	Hurler's Scheie's Hurler-Scheie compound	α-L-iduronidase	dermatan sulphate heparan sulphate
II A II B	Hunter's Hunter's mild	iduronate sulphatase	dermatan sulphate heparan sulphate
III A III B	Sanfilippo's A Sanfilippo's B	heparan sulphate sulphamidase α-N-acetylglucos-aminidase	heparan sulphate heparan sulphate
IV	Morquio's	α-N-acetylgalactos-amine-6-sulphatase	keratan sulphate
V	Vacant		
VI A VI B	Maroteaux-Lamy Maroteaux-Lamy (Mild)	N-acetylgalactosamine-4-sulphatase	dermatan sulphate
VII	β-glucuronidase deficiency (Sly's syndrome)	β-glucuronidase	dermatan sulphate heparan sulphate

Table 8/1 Summary of types of mucopolysaccharidosis

Neimann-Pick disease

In this condition there is an abnormal accumulation of a compound called sphingomyelin due to the absence of the enzyme sphingomyelinase. There are probably five different clinical forms of this condition but the commonest is the infantile form.

During the first six months of life there may be a history of early persistent jaundice and later failure to thrive, feeding difficulties, recurrent vomiting and bouts of fever, together with a protuberant abdomen due mainly to hepato-splenomegaly. A chest x-ray will reveal widespread pulmonary infiltration with the storage compound. Progressive deterioration after the age of six months is associated with hypotonia and possibly cerebellar disorders; a cherry-red spot is seen at the macula in about a quarter of cases, and occasionally fits occur.

A blood film may show vacuolated lymphocytes because of sphingomyelin accumulation within the cells. In the bone marrow large *foam cells* are found, which are an accumulation of sphingomyelin. The diagnosis may ultimately be confirmed by detecting low or absent levels of sphingomyelinase in the white cells. Antenatal diagnosis is possible.

Neimann-Pick disease is autosomally recessively inherited and like Tay-Sachs disease is more common in Ashkenazim Jews. It is occasionally referred to as an *amaurotic familial idiocy*.

Gaucher's disease

There is an abnormal storage of cerebrosides in Gaucher's disease owing to a deficiency of the enzyme glucocerebrosidase. Two clinical forms exist: a chronic form in which the central nervous system seems to be largely unaffected, and an acute infantile form in which there is marked cerebral involvement.

ACUTE INFANTILE

These children are usually healthy until the age of four months, when they cease to thrive and develop a large abdomen, partly due to hepato-splenomegaly. They are anaemic, often develop a squint and rapidly deteriorate with misery, a whining cry, opisthotonic posturing, spasticity and progressive bulbar paresis. Death occurs at about the age of 12 months.

In the plasma there is often an elevated level of acid phosphatase due, in part, to the high body content of cerebrosides. In the bone marrow there are large cells, characteristic of this disorder and similar to, but not the same as, those found in Neimann-Pick disease. Liver biopsy will assist in establishing a definitive diagnosis but the more ready method of measuring enzyme levels in the white blood cells is the confirmatory investigation of choice.

Gaucher's disease is autosomally recessively inherited and antenatal diagnosis is possible.

Batten's disease (neuronal ceroid lipofuscinosis)

There are known to be four clinical forms of this disorder, in which there is intraneuronal storage of a lipofuscin material. The exact defect in these disorders is unknown. The compound stored is normally found in nervous tissue as part of an ageing process. No enzyme abnormality has yet been identified.

INFANTILE BATTEN'S DISEASE (SANTAVOURI OR FINNISH TYPE)

Marked deterioration is noted by the age of one year, with the development of mental retardation, microcephaly, ataxia, visual loss, and myoclonic jerks. During the third year the disease enters a quiescent phase but death will occur by the age of six years.

LATE INFANTILE BATTEN'S DISEASE (JANSKY-BIELSCHOWSKY)

Seizures, often myoclonic, are one of the earliest signs of this form of Batten's disease, which commences between the ages of eighteen months and four years. The seizures become more severe, and ataxia, progressive mental deterioration, visual loss, and optic atrophy also develop. Jansky-Bielschowsky disease has sometimes been referred to as a *late infantile amaurotic familial idiocy*. Death is before the age of 10 years.

JUVENILE BATTEN'S DISEASE (SPIELMEYER-VOGT)

The onset is between the age of six and 10 years with progressive visual loss due to retinitis pigmentosa. Following the onset of the visual disorder, mental deterioration will occur with, later, seizures, ataxia, swallowing difficulties, rigidity, and spastic quadriplegia. Death will occur in patients with Spielmeyer-Vogt disease between the ages of 15 and 25 years.

There is an adult form of Batten's disease known as Kuf's disease, in which, at about puberty, a non-specific psychological disturbance develops with later mental deterioration together with a cerebellar disorder. The visual signs in this condition are not as marked as in the other forms of Batten's disease. The course may be prolonged, extending over some 20 years.

Investigations

The investigations of the different forms of Batten's disease will be considered together.

White blood cells show a high incidence of vacuolated lymphocytes in the Spielmeyer-Vogt variety of Batten's disease and also the late infantile Jansky-Bielschowsky form. The electroencephalogram (EEG) in the Santavouri variety shows a progressive slowing and diminution of the brain waves. This will be noted with the aid of serial recordings. In the Jansky-Bielschowsky form, slow photic stimulation will produce very high amplitude discharges in the EEG over the occipital lobes. An electroretinogram (ERG) shows reduced or absent responses in all forms of Batten's disease because of the degeneration of the superficial layers of the retina.

The lipofuscin material will be stored in neuronal plexi of the gastro-intestinal tract as well as in the brain. Therefore, as an alternative to a brain biopsy a rectal biopsy can be used to demonstrate this material in the nervous tissue. The pattern of storage varies between the different forms of Batten's disease, and the varieties may be distinguished from each other by their staining reactions. Electron microscopic examination of skin and marrow samples has disclosed various inclusion bodies which may also be diagnostic of the conditions and differentiate one from the other.

All the forms of Batten's disease are autosomally recessively inherited, but unfortunately no method of antenatal diagnosis yet exists.

SUB-ACUTE ENCEPHALOPATHY (SUB-ACUTE SCLEROSING PANENCEPHALITIS (SSPE))

This is a central nervous system degenerative disorder in which a measles-like virus is found in the brain. The onset may be insidious, being several months to years after an attack of typical measles.

Intellectual deterioration, personality change, and ultimately 'myoclonic jerking' are the principal features on presentation. The disease progresses relentlessly into spasticity, profound dementia with cortical blindness, and seizures which are difficult to control; death is inevitable.

The EEG will, at least at some point in the illness, show some characteristic changes. Regularly recurring paroxysms of polyspikes, together with a generally abnormal record, is diagnostic of SSPE. The cerebrospinal fluid has an elevated titre to the measles virus and changes in the protein content of the fluid are detected by performing a colloidal gold (Lange's) test.

DEGENERATIVE DISORDERS (WITHOUT STORAGE)

In some neurodegenerative disorders no biochemical basis for the disorder has yet been identified and there is no evidence of abnormal storage material or the presence of a virus. Two examples are included in this chapter and two others, ataxia-telangiectasia and Freidreich's ataxia, are described in Chapter 15.

Dystonia musculorum deformans

This progressive disorder is characterised by slow spasmodic twisting and turning of the spine and limbs. Changes in brain structure have been described but the cause is unknown.

There are two forms of dystonia musculorum deformans. An autosomal recessive form, more common in Ashkenazim Jews, has its onset in childhood and initially rapidly increases in severity; the autosomal dominant form which is not more common in Jews, has a highly variable age of onset.

The initial symptoms in both forms are similar, with slow

writing movements of a foot, a hand, the neck or trunk. The duration and frequency of the movements gradually increases until ultimately the abnormal postures are fixed. In the earlier stages the movements and abnormal postures disappear in sleep. In the autosomal recessive form the abnormal movements are more common in the limbs, while in the dominant form they are more common in the trunk and neck.

The condition has to be distinguished from the dystonia that is part of cerebral palsy and also from Wilson's disease (see Chapter 9). Frequently patients are diagnosed as having an hysterical illness, partly because of the bizarre postures in the absence of objective neurological signs.

Treatment is difficult. A number of muscle relaxant drugs may be helpful for a time; so-called stereotactic surgery may be helpful in some patients, especially those in whom the problems are confined to one side of the body. The overall prognosis is not good and most patients suffer increasing disability.

Huntington's chorea

The principal features of this condition are progressive chorea and mental deterioration, predominantly with onset in adulthood. The disease is dominantly inherited.

Atrophy of the part of the brain known as the caudate nucleus, and catecholamine abnormalities are well described. The cause is unknown.

In about two per cent of cases the onset may be in early childhood and in most of these the transmission will be from the father.

The clinical picture in childhood onset of Huntington's chorea is predominantly one of mental deterioration, rigidity and later the development of seizures. Still later the chorea characteristic of adult form appears.

Diagnosis is greatly supported by a positive family history which is present in virtually all cases. There is no effective treatment.

The late onset of the disorder—often not until the fourth or fifth decade, and the absence of a means of preclinical diagnosis render genetic counselling a very difficult task.

This chapter has described only some of the neurodegenerative disorders in childhood, all of which are fortunately rare. Despite knowing the biochemical basis for most of these disorders, few have so far proved amenable to treatment. Attempts have been made to replace missing enzymes, diets of various sorts have been attempted, and methods of decreasing the levels of the abnormally stored material have also been attempted.

The care of a child with a degenerative disorder places great demands on those professionals involved and calls for a very special form of support for the parents. Parental feelings may often include anger that there is no specific treatment—an anger often directed at the medical and other caring professions. Parents may feel that it is their fault that they have a child with such a disorder. This parental reaction is not unique and is recognised in many parents whose children are handicapped.

The detection of an enzyme deficiency in several neurodegenerative disorders, the development of modern tissue culture techniques for growing cells and modern techniques for amniocentesis have fortunately allowed the diagnosis of several of these disorders to be made in early pregnancy in those mothers who have had an affected child. Termination of that pregnancy can then be offered if it is shown that the pregnancy will result in a similarly affected offspring. This aspect of management is vitally important for those parents with a child with a neurodegenerative disorder, because so many of the diseases are autosomally recessively inherited and the chance of recurrence high.

FURTHER READING

Gordon, N. (1976). *Paediatric Neurology for the Clinician*. Spastics International Medical Publications. Clinics in Developmental

Medicine No 59/60. William Heinemann Medical Books Ltd, London.

Jabbour, J. T. et al (1973). *Paediatric Neurology Handbook.* Henry Kimpton Publishers, London.

Menkes, J. H. (1980). *Textbook of Child Neurology*, 2nd edition. Lea and Febiger Co, Philadelphia.

9. Disorders of metabolism—the effects on brain function

The nervous system is highly sensitive to metabolic and biochemical dysfunction. High or low blood levels of various substances can cause long-term effects on the brain and nervous tissue. In the previous chapter those diseases caused by the presence of additional substances in the brain and also those caused by nonspecific degeneration of brain function were discussed. In this chapter the disorders in which brain damage may occur from abnormal blood levels of various substances are considered.

The first group of these disorders are those due to temporary alteration in body biochemistry; for example, hypoglycaemia, hypocalcaemia, and other electrolyte disturbances. The second group are biochemical abnormalities consequent upon differing forms of *inborn errors of metabolism*. Examples of inborn errors of amino acid, urea, purine, carbohydrate, thyroid gland, and copper metabolism will be briefly described.

In children presenting with neurological disorders, particularly seizures, variable mental dysfunction, or other intermittent changes, the possibility of a metabolic cause should be considered. In some, such biochemical abnormalities may be easily remediable, but in others highly complex management is required.

HYPOGLYCAEMIA

The premature or 'small-for-dates' infant is particularly at risk from hypoglycaemia, which in the past has been strongly implicated in the aetiology of cerebral diplegia. Hypoglycaemia is a preventable disorder if everyone who attends the newborn is aware of it and actively seeks it out. This is now easily done with

Dextrostix estimations on finger or heel prick blood samples, and laboratory facilities are not necessary. Any minor twitching or jitteriness in a neonate should be suspected as being due to hypoglycaemia. Treatment is usually the provision of extra sugar. Hypoglycaemia should be suspected in the neonate and in other infants who present with seizures. This is an eminently preventable cause of serious brain damage but good results depend on early recognition and treatment.

HYPOCALCAEMIA

This is not uncommonly seen in neonates who are otherwise healthy and who are bottle fed, typically at about five days old. It may also be seen in the sick infant, particularly those with diarrhoea. Hypocalcaemia may be sufficiently strongly suspected that oral calcium may be given without necessarily checking the serum level. The outlook if treatment is appropriate and early is good.

Other electrolyte disturbances may be seen in neonates and young infants, particularly when ill, e.g. low or high blood sodium (hypo and hypernatraemia), low magnesium (hypomagnesaemia), and also other acid-base disturbances. The giving of artificial feeds as opposed to breast milk inevitably increases the risks of many of these biochemical disorders. High-solute feeds increase the risk of hypernatraemia in the presence of even a mild viral infection.

An interesting but rare biochemical disorder that will present in the neonatal period as severe seizures is pyridoxine (vitamin B_6) dependency. High doses of pyridoxine, perhaps given intravenously, will rapidly stop the seizures and development will subsequently be normal. This disorder is not really understood, but as pyridoxine is a *co-enzyme* its administration may facilitate the 'opening up' of certain metabolic pathways. In an infant in whom there is no definite explanation for seizures, a therapeutic trial of pyridoxine should be considered. If this diagnosis is missed, not only will the seizures continue but brain damage will occur and the later administration of pyridoxine will not produce any response. Interestingly, mothers of children with pyridoxine dependency describe what sound very much like intra-uterine seizures.

INBORN ERRORS OF AMINO ACID METABOLISM

There are a number of inborn errors of amino acid metabolism, all of which are recessively inherited. In some of these, speculation exists as to whether the abnormality is purely a biochemical phenomenon or a definite disorder, for example, *histidinaemia*, which is due to a defect in the enzyme histidase; others are almost always associated with definite clinical disorders. Three of the more common inborn errors of amino acid metabolism will be discussed.

Phenylketonuria

This is the most well-known inborn error of amino acid metabolism in the United Kingdom and Europe. In this disorder there is a high level of phenylalanine and a low level of tyrosine in the body due to the deficiency or absence of the enzyme phenylalanine hydrolase. The approximate incidence of this disorder in the United Kingdom is between one in 7 000 and one in 10 000 births. If untreated, phenylketonuria can be expected to be associated in virtually all cases with severe mental retardation, microcephaly, and seizures. A severe eczematous rash is often seen in the untreated infant, as well as a fair complexion. The diagnosis of phenylketonuria can be made as early as the fifth to seventh day after birth in a child with a normal protein intake, using the Guthrie microbiological technique applied to a small sample of blood obtained from a heel prick. All newborn babies in the United Kingdom are screened in this way. The disorder is treatable with a low phenylalanine diet. Phenylalanine is an essential amino acid and, therefore, the levels in the blood need to be monitored, i.e. the level must be normal and not absent. In principle the diet is adjusted so that the total source of amino acids is from a casein hydrolysate from which phenylalanine has been removed by adsorption onto charcoal. With careful dietary management in childhood normal development can virtually be assured.

More recently it has been realised that although the biochemical features of phenylketonuria may be present the clinical features may not. As total population screening has only been achieved for approximately 15 years, there are several unknown 'biochemically phenylketonuric' adults with no obvious signs of the disease. Women with raised phenylalanine levels cause concern because it is now recognised that there is an increased risk of these mothers producing babies with congenital abnormalities. Such babies may have a syndrome which includes microcephaly, mental retardation and other neurological disorders. Children with phenylketonuria treated with a low phenylalanine diet are seldom maintained on this after the age of 15 and many stop much earlier with no obvious adverse effects to themselves. It remains a dilemma as to whether all mothers should be screened antenatally for high levels of phenylalanine and whether termination should be automatically offered. It is not known if putting the mother on a special diet will decrease the risk of, or prevent the occurrence of, fetal abnormalities.

A mother of a child with a neurological abnormality for which there is no obvious explanation should have her amino acid concentrations checked as she might be a biochemical, but clinically unaffected, phenylketonuric. Counselling can then be offered.

Maple syrup urine disease

This is so named because of the smell of the urine. The condition is due to a high level of leucine, isoleucine, and valine secondary to a defect in oxidative decarboxylation of the branched chain amino acids.

The most common clinical picture is of severe neurological deterioration preceded by respiratory irregularity and opisthotonic posturing and death occurring within a month of birth. More recently, other forms of this condition have been described with intermittent ataxia, acidosis, and drowsiness; and another form in which there is moderate mental retardation only.

It is possible, although difficult, to treat maple syrup urine disease with a synthetic diet, using the same principles as with phenylketonuria.

Antenatal diagnosis is feasible, using cultured fibroblasts obtained after amniocentesis; such testing can be offered to mothers who have already produced a child with this condition.

Homocystinuria

Elevated levels of homocystine and depressed levels of cystine occur in this disorder, due to decreased activity of the enzyme cystathionine synthetase. Affected children are tall and thin and often blonde with erythematous skin. Ultimately the lenses of the eye dislocate and there is also a high incidence of recurrent thrombosis. Mental retardation is common, together with seizures and spasticity; all are thought to be due to the thrombosis.

The diagnosis, apart from on clinical grounds, is made by measuring urinary and plasma homocystine and cystine levels.

Some patients benefit from the early administration of vitamin B_6, in others a high cystine and low methionine diet has been claimed to be helpful, while in others neither of these seems to produce any benefit.

ABNORMALITIES OF THE KREBS' UREA CYCLE

The fundamental pathway converting ammonia into urea can have a number of inborn errors. While the detailed biochemistry differs, each of the five forms currently known may share the common biochemical abnormality of a high blood ammonia (arginosuccinic aciduria, citrullinaemia, ornithine transcarbamoylase deficiency, carbamoyl phosphate synthetase deficiency, and lysine intolerance).

Vomiting, often early in infancy, is usually the earliest sign of any of the abnormalities of the Krebs' urea cycle and will be related to protein ingestion. As well as this, mental dysfunction, neurological signs and seizures frequently occur. In many of these disorders the infants do not survive; indeed ornithine trans-carbamoylase deficiency, which is X linked, is fatal in affected males in the neonatal period so that the condition in real terms is seen only in heterozygote females. In a number of these disorders much milder forms exist, giving rise to various neurological symptoms. The relationship to protein ingestion is interesting and occasionally it will be noted that affected individuals avoid food that is high in protein.

INBORN ERRORS OF PURINE METABOLISM

The Lesch–Nyhan syndrome is an X-linked disorder of purine metabolism in which hyperuricaemia develops due to a deficiency or absence of the enzyme hypoxanthine-guanine phosphoribosyl transferase (HG-PRT). This deficiency or absence can be demonstrated using blood cell preparations and cultured fibroblasts. The clinical picture is that of initial normality and then towards the end of the first year of life mental retardation is apparent, as are choreo-athetosis, spasticity, aggressiveness, and compulsive self-mutilation which causes the child to gnaw away at the lips and fingertips.

The high uric acid inevitably gives rise to a renal disease of a type normally associated with gout, but seldom is there any evidence of this latter disorder. Mothers of such boys may have high uric acid levels particularly postmenopausally. Antenatal diagnosis with estimation of HG-PRT in fibroblasts from the amniotic fluid is possible.

Treatment is ineffective, although the use of the drug allopurinol can ameliorate the renal complications which are often the cause of death.

High blood levels of uric acid may be seen in infants of either sex with mental retardation but with normal HG-PRT activity;

while the clinical picture may be remarkably similar to Lesch–Nyhan syndrome the enzyme abnormality has yet to be identified.

INBORN ERRORS OF CARBOHYDRATE METABOLISM

Galactosaemia is an inborn error of carbohydrate metabolism in which there is an intolerance to lactose and galactose owing to an absence of the enzyme galactose-l-phosphate uridyl transferase. Galactose-l-phosphate accumulates and the clinical picture may be one of vomiting, failure to thrive, diarrhoea, persistent neonatal jaundice with, soon after the neonatal period, the development of hepato-splenomegaly, cataracts, hypotonia, and later mental retardation. There are known to be several differing sub-groups of this disorder with varying severity.

The diagnosis should be suspected from the clinical picture and the finding of a reducing sugar in the urine. Paper chromatography will identify the sugar and an absolute diagnosis can be made from the red cell estimation of galactose-l-phosphate uridyl transferase.

The withdrawal of milk and the institution of lactose-free food such as Nutramigen is curative. The liver disorder is halted and the cataracts may disappear.

Antenatal diagnosis is possible by enzyme estimation and thought has been given to neonatal screening. At present too many false positive results occur for screening to be practical.

THYROID DEFICIENCY

Evidence has accumulated that congenital hypothyroidism (low thyroid function) may be twice as common as phenylketonuria in the United Kingdom. Furthermore, encouraging results have been obtained from the very early treatment of affected infants. Without treatment, growth and mental development is severely compromised.

Techniques have now been refined that enable thyroid function to be easily assessed at birth by the measurement of the level of thyroid stimulating hormone (TSH) on very small samples of blood. Several centres have now incorporated this into their routine screening of the newborn.

WILSON'S DISEASE (HEPATOLENTICULAR DEGENERATION)

This inborn error of copper metabolism is associated with cirrhosis of the liver and degenerative changes in the basal ganglia of the brain. There is a low level or even absence of caeruloplasmin (a copper-binding protein) in the blood. Deposition of copper in many tissues and the development of cupricuria (high levels of copper in the urine) occur. It is this copper deposition in the basal ganglia of the brain, liver, kidneys, and cornea that accounts for the clinical signs. The exact cause of the disease is not known, although many argue that it is due to the low level or absence of caeruloplasmin.

Wilson's disease in childhood more commonly presents as a liver disorder. When neurological symptoms develop it is usually in the older child or adolescent; the first signs are often bulbar with indistinct speech and difficulty in swallowing. A tremor may occur and become severe and generalised, as a clinical picture reminiscent of Parkinson's disease develops. There will be a deposition of copper in the eye which gives rise to the diagnostic sign of Kayser–Fleischer rings in which a brown deposit can be seen in front of the iris when using a slit lamp.

Investigations in these patients reveal a very low level of caeruloplasmin or its total absence, a very high urinary excretion of copper, abnormal liver function tests, an excessive amount of amino acids in the urine, and the Kayser–Fleischer rings.

Wilson's disease is treatable with D-penicillamine, which is a chelating agent able to remove the excess copper from the body. A low copper diet is also instituted. Treatment is life-long and as the disorder is autosomally recessively inherited there may be other members of the family who are biochemically affected but at the time are asymptomatic. These family members should be identified and offered therapy before their symptoms develop. Metabolic disorders that are highly relevant to nervous system function are continually being 'discovered'. In any child with a neurological disorder that may have a biochemical and metabolic basis there is a need for a very careful evaluation. In some cases the effects of the disorder may be modified with either special diets, as in phenylketonuria and galactosaemia, or the use of co-enzymes as in some cases of homocystinuria; or treated with a drug such as that used in Wilson's disease. The success of phenyl-ketonuria screening and considerable experience with screening for congenital hypothyroidism also raises the question of total population screening for other metabolic disorders, given that there is a reliable, cheap test and an effective treatment for the condition.

FURTHER READING

Stanbury, J. B., Wyngaarden, J. B. and Frederickson, D. S. (1979). *The Metabolic Basis of Inherited Disease*, 4th edition. McGraw-Hill, New York.

THE EFFECT OF EXTERNAL FACTORS ON NERVOUS SYSTEM FUNCTION

10. Infections of the nervous system

It is important to be aware of the immediate and long-term effects which may ensue from infection and inflammation of the central nervous system. In this chapter some of the effects of central nervous system infection and inflammation will be discussed in relation to intact but developing nervous tissue. Reference has already been made to the greater susceptibility to infection of children with structural abnormalities of the brain and spinal cord. In Chapter 11 the increased risk of infection after severe head injury is discussed.

Infective or inflammatory conditions of the nervous system can be considered as either affecting the meninges and cerebrospinal fluid (CSF), the central nervous system tissue itself (the brain and spinal cord), or the peripheral nerves.

Meningitis is an infection of the meningeal coverings of the brain and spinal cord; *encephalitis* is an infection of the brain substance itself; *myelitis* is an inflammation or infection of the spinal cord. Overlap is common in these three conditions. With meningitis there is often at least some inflammation and infection of the brain substance and when this is marked the term *meningo-encephalitis* is used. Furthermore, there is sometimes evidence of inflammation and infection of both the brain and spinal cord and here the description *encephalo-myelitis* is used. A severe focal infection of the brain substance can cause abscess formation—a cerebral abscess.

Conditions which affect the peripheral nervous tissue such as tetanus and poliomyelitis will not be described. Both these conditions, although they still occur, are rare in the United Kingdom. The importance of active immunisation programmes is obvious in maintaining this rarity.

In central nervous system infection the infecting organism must be identified so that treatment is effective. In bacterial meningitis microscopy and culture of the CSF will usually identify the organism. Special techniques have to be used to identify the virus causing a viral meningitis or encephalitis. Such viral studies may be inconclusive, and blood tests showing the presence of a rising antibody titre are needed to confirm the diagnosis. The development of a neurological symptom after an acute systemic infection such as measles is well recognised, and in such situations the only evidence of viral involvement will be a high antibody titre specific to the virus responsible for the preceding infection.

MENINGITIS

The clinical picture will vary according to the infecting organism and the age of the child. Nevertheless, there are some features of meningitis that might be considered as typical and relatively specific.

There will often be a generalised illness which will vary in severity. In the older child obvious headaches and irritability —often with pyrexia, photophobia, and neck stiffness—will strongly suggest the diagnosis of meningitis. In the younger child a bulging fontanelle may be seen when the meningitis is severe. Inflammation of the meningeal coverings of the brain will cause pain with movements that stretch the meninges. The patient will attempt to limit these movements or complain of significant discomfort. This situation can be demonstrated when a supine patient with meningitis has the hip flexed and the knee extended. The movement of the leg will be resisted by the patient and will cause significant pain. This is known as Kernig's sign. By a similar mechanism, passive flexion of the patient's neck will produce active flexion of the legs. This is Brudzinski's sign. What can sometimes be confusing diagnostically is the patient who has a stiff neck but no other signs to suggest meningitis. This is known as *meningism* and can be seen in such different diseases as lobar pneumonia, a posterior cervical lymphadenopathy, or a pharyngitis.

Investigations of a patient with meningeal signs consist of a blood count and a lumbar puncture. An abnormal blood count may suggest the presence of an infection. As meningitis is often part of a more generalised infective process such as a septicaemia, blood cultures are important. The definitive diagnosis is by examination of the CSF obtained by lumbar puncture. A lumbar puncture must not be attempted in the presence of raised intracranial pressure.

In bacterial meningitis the CSF, instead of being clear, may be very cloudy due to the presence of an increased amount of protein and inflammatory cells. The inflammatory cells in a bacterial meningitis are usually polymorphonuclear leucocytes, whereas in viral meningitis, tuberculous meningitis and the later stages of a bacterial meningitis (possibly already partially treated) the cells are mononuclear leucocytes. With any infection or inflammation, but most particularly with bacterial infections, the protein content of the CSF is likely to be increased.

The level of glucose in the CSF is lowered in a bacterial infection and most particularly in tuberculosis, when it may be virtually unmeasurable. Normal levels will be found in viral meningitis and in encephalitis. With the younger child it is important that the level of sugar in the CSF is compared to that in the blood because hypoglycaemia may be present, so rendering the CSF glucose level difficult to assess.

In most cases of bacterial meningitis the infecting organism may be identified, except when antibiotics have already been used. Bacteria are identified by their general shape, morphology, and staining reactions; the most common staining reaction being Gram's stain, with which a large number of the bacteria that cause meningitis can be classified as being either Gram-negative or Gram-positive. If tuberculous meningitis is suspected then an entirely different staining technique is used—the Ziehl–Neelsen method.

Cerebrospinal fluid is always inoculated into a culture medium so the exact nature of the organism can be determined, together with its antibiotic sensitivity. If tuberculosis is suspected a different culture medium has to be used. Viruses require specialised culture techniques.

As well as examination of the CSF there are a number of other ancillary investigations which may be helpful such as chest x-rays, skin tests for tuberculosis, and swabs taken from the nose and rectum for bacteria and virus isolation.

Bacterial meningitis

Bacterial meningitis is a serious illness with a significant mortality despite the improvements in therapy in recent years and the employment of better and more powerful antibiotics. Complications that can follow meningitis include communicating hydrocephalus due to adhesions around the exit foramina of the ventricular system in the posterior fossa, focal neurological deficits, cranial nerve lesions, mental handicap, behavioural disorders, and epilepsy. Early diagnosis and energetic treatment is associated with the most favourable outcome.

The following are the most commonly encountered meningitides in the United Kingdom.

HAEMOPHILUS INFLUENZAE MENINGITIS

Infection with this Gram-negative organism is most common in the younger child below the age of five years, although it is rare below the age of three months. The onset of the illness is insidious with non-specific features suggesting a simple upper respiratory tract infection. Within a few days the more specific features of meningitis will appear. Examination of the CSF will give the characteristic findings associated with bacterial meningitis.

Treatment is with high doses of ampicillin (Penbritin) and/or chloramphenicol (Chloromycetin) or other antibiotics shown to be appropriate after sensitivity testing of the organism.

While the complications of meningitis referred to previously occur with Haemophilus meningitis there is a higher than usual chance of the development of subdural effusions and occasionally a cerebral abscess, both of which require specific treatment, once diagnosed.

The mortality of this condition is about 20 per cent and in those that survive up to 30 per cent may have some neurological sequelae.

MENINGOCOCCAL MENINGITIS

This is sometimes still referred to as *cerebrospinal fever*. This form of meningitis can affect almost any age group. It was well known for its tendency to occur in epidemics, particularly in dry conditions and with crowded accommodation as in some schools and army barracks. In the United Kingdom large epidemics are now rare, although there can still be a tendency for small outbreaks to occur within specified areas.

The meningococcus is a Gram-negative organism that can be carried in the nose by asymptomatic individuals. Transmission is usually by inhalation, although the degree of infectivity is uncertain. There is often a preceding non-specific illness but the onset of the meningitis is acute. Some patients will be desperately ill and collapse within a few hours. As well as the clinical features of a meningitis or a septicaemia, this disorder is further characterised by typical skin lesions known as *petechiae*. Petechiae are caused by small subcutaneous bleeds and may appear as small individual spots or coalesce to form bruise-like lesions. One of the first places for these to occur is within the inferior conjunctiva. In a severely ill patient the skin lesions may be severe and the petechiae coalesce in places to form large necrotic areas. The CSF findings are those of a bacterial meningitis, and blood culture will grow the meningococcus.

It is important to institute urgent treatment. This is usually by giving high doses of intravenous penicillin and, because of the collapsed state of many of the patients, high doses of steroids. In milder cases the outcome is excellent; where the child is collapsed the outlook for survival is not good. Unfortunately the latter occurs quite often.

With meningococcal infections complications can occur and include arthritis, encephalitis, heart failure, adrenal failure (sometimes known as Waterhouse–Friderichsen syndrome), and disseminated intravascular coagulation in which platelets sludge within the body tissues and cause a life-threatening bleeding disorder.

The need to treat asymptomatic carriers is a little controversial because the organism is probably of such low infectivity. Claims have been made that the antibiotic rifampicin can eradicate the organism in such cases.

PNEUMOCOCCAL MENINGITIS

This type of meningitis is usually a complication of an infection elsewhere, such as in an ear or the chest, or due to some structural defect or abnormality in the skull associated with a sinus from the skin through to the meninges. It is also described in some patients who have had the spleen removed, or in others who have a deficient immunological system.

The clinical picture is that of meningitis of fairly rapid onset; lumbar puncture will demonstrate the typical findings of a bacterial meningitis and the isolation of a Pneumococcus which is Gram-positive.

Treatment is with high doses of intravenous penicillin, to which the organism is always sensitive. The outlook after treatment is generally good. A possible underlying cause of the meningitis must be sought.

NEONATAL MENINGITIS

This is a very serious illness, which may have a non-specific clinical presentation. The specific signs of meningitis may be absent and the infant may simply appear to be generally unwell. The most common infective organisms in neonatal meningitis are probably the Gram-negative E. coli and Proteus. Ill and premature infants, and those for whom there was prolonged rupture of the membranes before delivery, are especially at risk. An 'infection screen' including examination of the CSF should be considered in any neonate who is unwell, failing to thrive, perhaps irritable, feeding poorly, pyrexial or hypothermic. Measurements of head circumference are important to detect the early development of hydrocephalus. Examination of the CSF is usually diagnostic but must be combined with a blood culture.

Treatment has to be started immediately and this may be before the definitive diagnosis of neonatal meningitis has been made. Powerful antibiotics in high doses are essential; blood levels of these drugs must be carefully monitored. A common combination of antibiotics is intravenous gentamicin and penicillin.

Mortality is high in this condition—between 60 and 70 per cent with 40 per cent of the survivors having some neurological sequelae. Hydrocephalus may develop in up to a third of the surviving children. Seizure disorders, mental retardation, and cerebral palsy may also result.

TUBERCULOUS MENINGITIS

This is a serious but treatable meningitis secondary to an often undiagnosed tuberculous infection elsewhere in the body. The onset is insidious, with a non-specific illness possibly stretching over many months. The signs of meningitis will ultimately present, often combined with evidence of raised intracranial pressure. Examination of the optic fundi may reveal tuberculous deposits in the retina of the eye. The CSF will contain a large number of mononuclear leucocytes and have an elevated level of protein but a low or absent level of glucose. Appropriate staining will be necessary to identify the organism. Chest x-rays may demonstrate a primary focus or miliary tuberculosis, although the focus of infection might be elsewhere in the body. Skin testing for tuberculosis with either the Mantoux or tine test may be negative. Treatment is with a combination of anti-tuberculous agents. These include sodium aminosalicylate (PAS), isoniazid, streptomycin, and rifampicin, possibly in combination with steroids. Steroids combined with antibiotics are used to reduce the risk of adhesions in the meninges, which produce hydrocephalus. Their use is controversial.

The mortality in tuberculosis is high—up to 40 per cent. There is significant morbidity, with the common occurrence of communicating hydrocephalus, and the incidence of neurological abnormalities in this group may be as high as 20 per cent.

Viral meningitis

To a greater extent than with bacterial infection there may be difficulty distinguishing between viral meningitis, encephalitis, or meningo-encephalitis.

Usually, viral meningitis is not a serious illness. The major diagnostic responsibility is not to confuse it with a bacterial illness. There is sometimes a clear association with a readily recognisable exanthem such as mumps, measles, rubella or varicella; whereas at other times there may be a rash and a gastro-intestinal illness suggestive of an enterovirus such as a Coxsackie virus.

The CSF findings are as described for bacterial meningitis, i.e. mononuclear leucocytes in the CSF, with a mildly elevated protein level, no organisms on microscopy, and a normal CSF sugar level. A virus may subsequently be grown from the CSF if it is appropriately cultured, although samples taken from rectal or nasal swabs are as likely to be productive diagnostically. The demonstration of a rising antibody titre to a virus over the course of the illness will confirm this as being the likely infecting organism.

The treatment of a viral meningitis is symptomatic. The outlook for complete recovery is normally good.

ENCEPHALITIS

The encephalitides are a group of disorders characterised by a combination of headache, drowsiness, alterations in consciousness, meningitic signs as described above and, with the more serious varieties, a significant generalised illness with deep coma, seizures, and respiratory arrest. There may be a definite relationship to a recognisable exanthem but, as with viral meningitis, it may be difficult clinically to identify the viral agent.

The CSF may be relatively normal or similar to that found in a viral meningitis. The electroencephalogram (EEG) may be helpful in demonstrating features associated with encephalitis. It is important to exclude the possibility of poisons, a cerebral abscess, hypertension, or a generalised metabolic disorder. Lead poisoning must be considered.

Herpes simplex encephalitis

This is usually, but not invariably, a severe encephalitis. In some there may be a typical herpetic skin lesion which obviously would be diagnostically helpful. Together with the generalised features of an encephalitis there may be signs that specifically suggest involvement of the temporal lobes of the brain, which may be so marked as to suggest a tumour.

In mild herpes simplex encephalitis no specific treatment is indicated but in the severe form intensive care therapy is essential. Support may be needed to control raised intracranial pressure and to assist respiration. Attempts have been made to treat this form of encephalitis with specific anti-viral agents but as yet the usefulness of these is still in some doubt.

The mortality is high. The outlook for survival must depend upon the severity of the infection, and in those that survive severe herpes simplex encephalitis there will be a high incidence of neurological sequelae.

CEREBRAL ABSCESS

In a child with a cerebral abscess the signs may develop acutely or insidiously over several weeks. The specific presentation may be with headache and vomiting, irritability, and signs suggesting raised intracranial pressure. Alteration in consciousness is common, although often fluctuating and, therefore, confusing. If the abscess is in the cerebellum there may be ataxia and difficulty with co-ordination. Children with cyanotic heart disease, whose blood may be polycythaemic and thickened, are at particular risk from developing abscesses. The mechanism is probably that of a small cerebral infarct caused by the polycythaemia being infected by a co-existing septicaemia. In other patients it is often difficult to identify the source of an infection, although otitis media, sinusitis, and an anatomical defect in the skull are sometimes causative.

If a cerebral abscess is strongly suspected clinically then a lumbar puncture is contra-indicated as this may produce significant shifts of the brain substance and the possibility of coning and respiratory arrest. When an abscess is suspected it is important that definitive neuro-radiological investigations are carried out. The investigation of choice would be a CAT scan; an EEG has some localising value in cases of cerebral abscess.

The treatment of a cerebral abscess is surgical. After localisation with a scan an attempt is made to cannulate the abscess cavity to produce some drainage of pus and to instil antibiotics. Very often a small amount of dye is placed in the abscess cavity so that the size can be seen on repeated skull x-rays. It also affords the opportunity to re-cannulate the abscess cavity if it is thought necessary. Most neurosurgeons take a conservative approach in treating a cerebral abscess which includes possible repeated cannulations and high doses of systemic antibiotics. Occasionally a primary excision of the abscess cavity is undertaken but the risks involved include significant brain scarring and an increased tendency to epilepsy.

This is still a serious condition with a high mortality. The earlier the diagnosis the better the outcome. Naturally if there is more than one abscess, which there can be, then the outlook is adversely affected. With cyanotic heart disease there may be multiple abscesses and consequently a poor prognosis.

MYELITIS

Myelitis implies a specific disease of the spinal cord, causing inflammation. Relationship to a virus infection may be tenuous and in some cases the lesion itself is undoubtedly a demyelination as in multiple sclerosis, but perhaps triggered by a virus infection.

The clinical picture is that of a disruption of the spinal cord at a specific level with weakness, absent tendon reflexes, paralysis of the bladder, and anaesthesia below the level of the myelitis. Pain may occur at the site of the lesion.

The CSF may be normal and an important responsibility diagnostically is to exclude compression of the spinal cord due to an abscess, a prolapsed intervertebral disc, or a tumour.

The use of steroids in the management of this condition is controversial; in most cases the outlook for a complete recovery without treatment over a period of weeks or months is good.

REYE'S SYNDROME (pronounced as in 'rye')

The relationship to a virus infection with this condition is again uncertain: reports do exist of epidemics of Reye's syndrome which appear to follow virus infections. There is also thought to be a particular association with a preceding varicella infection.

The onset is usually acute with a severe encephalitic illness and liver failure caused by fatty infiltration of the brain, liver, and also the kidneys. Apart from the findings of encephalitis, there may be high levels of ammonia and disturbance of blood clotting factors due to liver failure.

The outlook is often very poor and the only treatment that may be effective is that of exchange blood transfusions, or possibly repeated peritoneal dialyses.

ACUTE CEREBELLAR ATAXIA

This is a relatively common disorder in children which seems to occur after certain virus infections. The patients present with acute ataxia but minimal other signs of an encephalitis illness. It will be fully described in Chapter 15.

The CSF is usually normal or may show mild inflammatory changes, with a few white blood cells present.

The outlook is extremely good and the major initial diagnostic responsibility is, as with myelitis, to exclude a tumour or other lesion.

SUB-ACUTE SCLEROSING PANENCEPHALITIS (SSPE)

This condition is described on p. 114. The relationship with a previous measles infection, often months or years earlier, is well established.

SSPE is a degenerative disorder and has a characteristic clinical picture with mental deterioration over some weeks and then the ultimate development of seizures. Dementia follows.

There is a characteristic CSF picture with a high titre to a measles virus. A particularly abnormal EEG in which periodic high voltage electrical complexes are seen at regular intervals on the tracing is obtained at some stage during the illness. There is no treatment and death is inevitable.

In patients who have immunological impairment due either to neoplastic disease or to its treatment, a number of sub-acute encephalopathies similar to SSPE have been reported.

Viruses are almost certainly responsible for a wide range of neurological lesions, but the relationship is sometimes uncertain. Bell's palsy is often strongly suspected as being due to an inflammatory lesion of the facial nerve, caused by a virus infection. Herpes zoster is undoubtedly related to the same virus as that responsible for varicella. What is of particular interest to some research workers is the association between viral infections of the CNS and the ultimate development of conditions such as multiple sclerosis or other illnesses which are characterised by degeneration of the nervous system.

In this chapter an attempt has been made to outline the more common infective disorders of the central nervous system. These disorders are still serious even though in many cases the outlook has been revolutionised by modern antibacterial treatment.

Treatment of the more serious viral infections still awaits an effective therapeutic agent.

FURTHER READING

Illis, L. S. (Ed) (1975). *Viral Diseases of the Central Nervous System*. Baillière Tindall, London.

Warin, J. F., Ironside, A. G. and Mandal, B. K. (1979). *Lecture Notes on the Infectious Diseases*, 3rd edition. Blackwell Scientific Publications Limited, Oxford.

11. Injuries to the nervous system

Accidents to children are common. In the Western world accidental injury is the commonest cause of death between the ages of one and 14 years. Trauma to the central nervous system is the injury responsible for death in many. Knowledge of the circumstances of such accidents is important in providing a safe environment for children. The other causes of central nervous system trauma are non-accidental injury and birth injury.

Road traffic accidents are an obvious cause of central nervous system trauma whether the child is a pedestrian or a cyclist or a passenger within a car. Many children are exposed to road traffic unsupervised at an age when their predictability and reaction times are too immature. The wearing of seat belts is not as prevalent as might be desirable and children still travel in the front seats of cars. There are many other situations in which the inquisitive child is at risk, e.g. falling through a window, out of trees, or off apparatus; and young children may be hit by various playground objects, particularly swings. The prevention of the mortality and morbidity which is consequent upon head injuries is important. However, even with an active and successful programme of prevention in many of the situations described above 'bumps on the head' will inevitably remain common in active children.

HEAD INJURIES

Concussion is a term applied to a transient neural dysfunction resulting from trauma to the head and brain. Some alteration in the level of consciousness occurs and there will be amnesia for the moment of the accident and variable amnesia before (retrograde amnesia) and afterwards (post-traumatic). To some extent the severity and thus the likely outcome from such an injury is related to the length of retrograde amnesia. Young children with brain injuries appear to have a relatively greater capacity for recovery than older children and adults, because the elasticity of their skulls allows greater pressure distortion of the brain to occur. Children can suffer from *contre-coup* injury, which occurs when a blow to one side of the head causes the brain to impinge traumatically on the opposite side of the skull. The resulting signs and symptoms are therefore the result of injury to the opposite side of the head to that struck.

Head injuries may be *closed* or *open*. In open injuries the brain is exposed and is at risk of infection. Most head injuries in children are closed.

Management

The admission to hospital of the unconscious child or the child who has a history of unconsciousness of whatever length is essential. There is a need not only for careful observation to be carried out but also for an immediate assessment of the need for intervention. In many children a clear history of the severity of the head injury may be difficult to obtain. Poor memory of the event may reflect either unobserved loss of consciousness or the difficulty children have with recall. They may be pale and listless and vomit after a blow to the head, even without a period of loss of consciousness. To assess the severity of the injury, to detect early various complications which may need urgent treatment, and to ensure that recovery is satisfactory, children are usually admitted into hospital for a period of observation. The general principles governing observations in the case of a child admitted with a head injury are similar, whatever the severity.

At the time of initial presentation a thorough general as well as neurological examination is essential so that other injuries, whether recent or not so recent, may be detected. Shock must be treated. Scalp lacerations should be noted and, where necessary, sutured.

The level of responsiveness and consciousness should be carefully assessed and recorded. This will vary from full orientation to total unresponsiveness even to painful stimuli. Vital functions such as heart rate, respirations, and temperature control are dependent upon intact brain function, and records need to be kept of these.

Careful monitoring should continue at regular intervals using the initial signs as the baseline on which to measure improvement or deterioration. Monitoring will include an assessment of limb movement, vital function, pupil reaction, and response to commands. Of particular importance is the early detection of a collection of blood inside the skull which may present as a change in the reactivity of one pupil or other focal neurological signs.

Investigations

X-rays of the head are important, but not as important as full clinical assessment when a child is first brought to hospital. In many cases demonstration of the presence of a skull fracture does *not* indicate a need for any specific action. The presence of certain skull fractures, however, are very important because of their association with particular complications which include possible damage to the middle meningeal artery when a fracture of the parietal bone is seen; the risk of leakage of spinal fluid to the ear when the fracture extends to the base of the skull; and leakage of spinal fluid through the nose when a fracture involves the thin cribriform plate of the anterior fossa of the skull. The x-ray demonstration of a depressed skull fracture is important as some require surgical treatment at a later stage and a fracture of this type may indicate the presence of a penetrating injury.

In some circumstances more definitive radiological studies are required to investigate brain damage or the possible presence of collections of blood within the head. These include CAT or isotope scans and carotid angiograms.

Complications of head injury

Complications of head injury may occur soon after injury or much later; in the case of seizures, even up to four years after the initial trauma.

Cerebral oedema is a generalised swelling of the brain tissue which may develop some hours after brain injury and not begin to resolve until 48 hours later.

Management is by restriction of fluids, sometimes the use of steroids, ventilation on a respirator, diuretics, and very careful nursing care. What is sometimes seen is the inappropriate secretion of a hormone known as antidiuretic hormone (ADH), which can cause a generalised accumulation of body fluid and therefore even give rise to heart failure and congestion of the lungs.

An extradural haematoma is a collection of blood, often due to arterial bleeding (commonly of the middle meningeal artery). The sequence of events which is often described is that of a period of consciousness (lucid interval) after injury followed by fading consciousness with the possible development of a fixed pupil on the same side. This classic sequence, however, is relatively rare in children. Commonly there may be an increasing apathy, pallor and lack of movement of one side.

A need for rapid action is indicated. Evacuation of an extradural clot should take place immediately. Burr holes have to be made and the source of the bleeding identified. The bleeding may be arterial, in which case a large haematoma forms rapidly, or venous, when the haematoma may develop slowly as the result of an ooze. Seizures may occur.

A subdural haematoma is the result of bleeding below the dural layer covering the brain. After injury the subdural haematoma is usually associated with severe brain contusion and therefore the outlook is poor. However, a child may present with the signs and symptoms caused by the space-occupying effect of the subdural haematoma without a history of a very recent head injury. This is because some of these haematomata develop slowly and three weeks may separate the head injury, which might have been considered insignificant, and the presentation.

CEREBROSPINAL FLUID LEAKAGE

When a fracture gives rise to a leakage of spinal fluid through the nose this has to be considered a compound fracture. While both rhinorrhoea and otorrhoea in such cases cease within days, a special precaution has to be taken to prevent the risk of meningitis occurring by the use of antibiotics. If such leaks of spinal fluid are persistent a surgical repair of the defect is indicated, because of the serious risk of infection.

EPILEPSY

Seizures may occur at the time of injury as a result of the immediate effect of the trauma; those occurring 24 to 48 hours after injury are likely to be due to the effect of cerebral oedema or haematomata. The risk of seizures occurring is increased with penetrating injuries. When the first seizure occurs over a week after the injury the chance of repeated seizures is higher than when the first seizure occurs immediately associated with the injury. Patients may have their first seizures up to four years after the injury, because of brain scarring.

EMOTIONAL PROBLEMS

Recovery from a head injury obviously depends upon the severity of the initial trauma and whether any of the complications already referred to develop. Fortunately, most children will recover with no long lasting sequelae. However, various behavioural dysfunctions may persist for weeks or months in those in whom the injury may not have been very severe. This may be reflected in sleep disturbance, lethargy, poor school performance and a specific learning disorder, including the so-called 'post-traumatic syndrome'. In this, a few weeks or months after injury, periods of irritability, poor concentration and headaches may occur. The possibility of litigation, as in adults, may make the problem more pronounced.

VERTIGO

Intense and sudden onset of vertigo when the head is placed in certain positions may be either due to brainstem or inner ear damage. This relatively common problem after head injury is ultimately self-limiting.

MENTAL RETARDATION AND NEUROLOGICAL DEFICIT

Subsequent mental retardation and neurological deficit is more common after head injuries resulting in a period of coma of greater than 24 hours.

HYDROCEPHALUS

This may occasionally result from head injury and present as raised intracranial pressure. A shunting/bypass operation may be required.

GROWING FRACTURE

A child under three years who sustains a skull fracture, especially in the parietal region, may have a tear in the dural layer. An arachnoid cyst may eventually form through the defect, which will cause a gradual increase in separation of the fractured edges. This is the so-called 'growing fracture' and if not recognised will cause pressure on the underlying brain as well as a pulsating mass on the side of the skull. This rare complication, if recognised sufficiently early, may be rectified by surgery.

SPINAL CORD INJURIES

Injury to the spinal cord is commonly caused by falls (from any height), diving, and road traffic accidents (particularly whiplash injuries). It is usually a closed injury and fractures of cervical vertebrae 1, 2, 4, and 6 and thoracic vertebrae 10, 11, and 12 cause particular anxiety because damage to the underlying spinal cord at these levels can result in serious cord dysfunction. The severity of the injury is proportional to the amount of spinal cord damage.

In complete cord transection there will be anaesthesia, paralysis, loss of bladder and bowel function and tendon reflexes below the level of the injury. If the trauma is in the upper cervical region damage will occur which results in poor respiratory function and death will occur if artificial ventilation is not given. If the trauma is lower in the cervical region diaphragmatic breathing will be possible, for at least part of the nerve supply to the diaphragm will be intact.

Both during and after the acute phase, the nursing care of such patients is vitally important. Immediately after injury there may be spinal instability which needs evaluating; stabilisation may be required and can be achieved using surgery or traction. Severe muscle spasms may be present in the early phase after injury and need management. Because of the loss of voluntary control over bowel and bladder function special care is needed to prevent urinary infections and faecal impaction. Ultimately an automatic bladder develops so that pressure on the lower abdomen can be used regularly to achieve micturition. The bowels often need management with either laxatives and/or suppositories.

Severe cord injury is rarely reversible and after such injury children face life with permanent paralysis, often of the legs but in cases of neck injuries of all four limbs. If the injury is high in the cervical spine permanent assisted ventilation is required.

NON-ACCIDENTAL INJURY/BATTERED BABY SYNDROME

It is perhaps appropriate to consider this sadly not uncommon problem in this chapter as a large number of these infants do have significant head injuries.

Any child who presents with physical injuries for which there seems a poor explanation, or to which the parents' reaction appears abnormal, should be carefully examined by a doctor. In some the injury on full assessment is more severe than expected from the history.

Signs on examination of widespread bruising, scars from cigarette burns, and x-ray findings of various fractures in various states of healing may raise the possibility of repeated trauma or abuse. It must be remembered that violent shaking of a young child may produce severe brain injury without any external signs of bruising. It is vital that the possibility of child abuse is always considered, because if it is not recognised there is a tragically high mortality. Many children have a history of repeated injury, and checks need to be made as to whether there have been previous recorded injuries. Admission of any child about whom there is doubt is essential. Apart from attending directly to the child's medical needs and removing him from the risk of further injuries, careful consideration can then be given to the social problems and plans for the child's future care made.

PERINATAL TRAUMA

Extreme moulding of the head during labour can produce tearing of the veins within the dural linings of the skull which may result in slowly developing subdural haematomata, acute haemorrhage, or death. This problem is more common in the premature infant. Rarely, depressed fractures may occur because of the impingement of the fetal head against the pelvis or an incorrectly applied forceps blade. Such fractures are commonly associated with intracranial lesions. Cephalhaematoma, a lump on the head seen particularly after vacuum extraction, is a small collection of blood that lies between the outside of the skull bone and the periosteum, which is the layer of tissue closely applied to the bone. A linear fracture may lie underneath a cephalhaematoma. These lumps eventually disappear, though often leaving some calcification around their edges.

Breech deliveries can cause damage to the upper cervical cord, producing various clinical problems not dissimilar to those described above with cord trauma. Infants so affected may be erroneously diagnosed as having severe neuromuscular disease.

Damage to the brachial plexus that provides the nerve supply to the arm can also occur due to traction or to trauma. Trauma to the upper brachial plexus causes an Erb's palsy, in which the arm is internally rotated, adducted, extended at the elbow, and flexed at the wrist to give rise to the classic 'waiter's tip' position. When the lower brachial plexus is injured Klumpke's paralysis results, in which the arm tends to be somewhat flail-like and the hand is clawed. Associated with this may be a Horner's syndrome from damage to the sympathetic nerve chain that reaches down into the neck. With Horner's syndrome the eye may droop and there may be a small pupil on the affected side. Most plexus lesions have a good outlook and recovery usually takes place; nevertheless, referral for physiotherapy is fully justified.

Much perinatal trauma can be prevented by good, careful antenatal and obstetric care. Careful obstetric techniques performed by experienced staff undoubtedly diminish the incidence of damage to the brain from traumatic causes in the newly born infant.

FURTHER READING

Illingworth, C. M. (1978). *The Diagnosis and Primary Care of Accidents and Emergencies in Children: a Manual for the Casualty Officer and the Family Doctor*. Blackwell Scientific Publications Limited, Oxford.

Potter, J. M. (1974). *The Practical Management of Head Injuries*, 3rd edition. Lloyd Luke (Medical Books) Ltd, London.

Till, K. (1975). *Paediatric Neurosurgery for Paediatricians and Neurosurgeons*. Blackwell Scientific Publications Limited, Oxford.

NEOPLASTIC DISEASE OF THE NERVOUS SYSTEM

12. Brain tumours

Although brain tumours are uncommon in childhood they are, nevertheless, a significant cause of mortality in children over one year.

The presenting symptoms of a brain tumour are often non-specific and include a history of vomiting, intermittent headache, and listlessness. As these symptoms are often associated with many other childhood diseases a delay in achieving the correct diagnosis can result.

The vomiting, headache, and listlessness are the result of raised intracranial pressure (ICP) caused by the mass effect of the tumour. Raised ICP has many causes and associations and before describing childhood brain tumours it is essential to understand some of the mechanisms underlying raised ICP.

RAISED INTRACRANIAL PRESSURE

Intracranial pressure or the pressure within the cranial vault is a function of the size of the brain, the amount of cerebrospinal fluid (CSF) within and around the brain, and the amount of blood within the head. Minor increases in one may be compensated for by decreases in another. In the infant whose fontanelle has not closed and sutures not fused, an increase in pressure will cause an increase in head size. Any lesion that is big enough to exert a mass effect may produce increased pressure because of its size or, even if not large, interfere with CSF drainage by pressure on the ventricular system. There are many examples of such space-occupying lesions, including tumours, cerebral abscesses (Chapter 10), intracranial haematomata (Chapter 11), and large aneurysms (Chapter 5). Tumours are discussed in this chapter but some of the other major causes will be mentioned first because of their importance when considering the differential diagnosis of raised intracranial pressure.

Subdural haematomata and effusions, whether traumatic or infective in origin, will produce an increase in ICP and present as either increasing head size in the very young or markedly increased pressure in the older child.

A rare cause of raised ICP may be an overproduction of CSF due to a papilloma of the choroid plexus.

A further poorly understood cause is benign intracranial hypertension or pseudo-tumour cerebri. Here there appears to be a swelling of the brain that may be associated with the administration of certain drugs, e.g. tetracycline, high doses of vitamin A, or the rapid withdrawal of steroid medication. Although such associations do exist, in many patients no cause will be found. Diagnosis partly depends on the exclusion of a space-occupying lesion and treatment consists of large doses of steroids which are gradually reduced over a period of time, together sometimes with repeated lumbar punctures to remove CSF and decrease the ICP.

Raised ICP due to hydrocephalus is discussed in Chapter 4.

Diagnosis

The symptoms of raised ICP in children are dominated by headache and vomiting.

The headache is persistent but may vary in severity, often being worse in the morning. Children are often unable to localise the pain and describe it as being 'all over'. These severe headaches often produce a preference to lying still, as movement and crying aggravate the pain.

Vomiting is often associated with the headache of raised ICP and similarly may be more common in the morning and is not preceded or accompanied by nausea.

The important sign of raised ICP is papilloedema (swelling of the optic nerve or disc seen on examination with an ophthalmoscope). However, in the very young child whose skull is still able to expand this is an unusual finding. In some patients a squint may develop and the child may complain of double vision (due usually to paralysis of the sixth cranial nerve, which is responsible for the movement of the eye laterally). This nerve, after emerging from the brainstem, travels a long way within the skull and in the presence of increased pressure it may become pressed against the side of the tentorium. With very severe raised ICP there may be respiratory difficulties, slowing of the heart rate and a fall in blood pressure. These are due to compression of the vital centres in the brainstem.

Personality changes and listlessness are often described over a prolonged period in children with increasing ICP. In the presence of severely raised ICP this progresses to alterations in the level of consciousness and ultimately to coma.

Most brain tumours in children occur in the posterior fossa and raised ICP, due to pressure on the ventricular system, is an early sign. The presenting symptoms in at least half the patients include ataxia or unsteadiness because of the site of the tumour. Theoretically, ataxia should have some localising value but in practice this is not always so. Any of the signs and symptoms already referred to may be absent in a child with raised ICP but it would be unusual for all of them to be absent.

Investigations

The investigation of a child thought to have a tumour will include a complete physical examination, measurement of blood pressure, and plain skull x-rays.

An x-ray of the skull in a child with raised ICP will, in the young child, show distension of the sutures of the skull. In the older child with long-standing raised ICP the x-ray may show increased skull indentation from the brain—'copper beating'—and erosion of the posterior clinoid processes of the pituitary fossa. In some specific space occupying lesions other features may be apparent, such as calcification with a tumour or erosion of certain bony areas.

The investigations that follow will usually include a CAT scan. In some it may be necessary to proceed to angiographic studies and tomographic x-rays. With the modern development of neuroradiological techniques—particularly the CAT scan—the EEG has a limited place in the investigation of a child with raised ICP and a possible tumour.

A lumbar puncture should never be performed when a tumour is suspected as the sudden change in pressure below the mass may induce the brainstem to herniate through the foramen magnum and cause *coning*. This is something that is usually fatal as the vital centres that control heart rate and respiration are compromised.

VARIETIES OF BRAIN TUMOUR

Most tumours of childhood are not only situated in the posterior fossa but are also of glial origin, i.e. arising from central nervous system tissue. These tumours may be cerebellar astrocytomas—often low grade and cystic—medulloblastomas, or ependymomas. Tumours of the choroid plexus, optic pathways, the pineal gland, the pituitary gland, and craniopharyngiomas are relatively less common.

Medulloblastoma

This is the commonest intracranial tumour of childhood and may occur at any time during the first decade of life, most commonly in the first half. Theories exist that the medulloblastoma originates from *rests* of primitive cells of embryonal origin. Very often these cells appear to be within the roof of the fourth ventricle. This is often, therefore, a midline tumour—arising in the posterior fossa. Cells may become free in the CSF and the seeding of malignant cells may occur anywhere within the subarachnoid space.

The history of illness may be short, characterised by ataxia, neck stiffness, and the signs of raised ICP. The neck stiffness may suggest a diagnosis of meningitis. Patients with medulloblastomas are often particularly ill—more than might be expected from the length of the history.

Diagnosis is based upon the history and clinical examination, a CAT scan (see Fig. 3/5, p. 49) and possibly examination of the CSF for malignant cells. Final and certain diagnosis is dependent upon surgical exploration.

Treatment of these tumours is with a combination of surgical removal, which is never complete, and radiotherapy of the brain and spinal cord. More recently this has been combined with chemotherapy (anticancer drugs). Although dramatic improvements may result from radiotherapy, the long-term survival used to be very poor. Survival now appears to be more encouraging partly because of the improved use of radiotherapy and chemotherapy.

Astrocytoma of the cerebellum

This glial tumour of the cerebellum is one of the commonest brain tumours in children. Rarely, similar tumours occur in the cerebral hemispheres.

Cerebellar astrocytomas vary greatly in the degree of their malignancy. Many are at least partially cystic and the tumour as a whole separates readily from the remaining cerebellar hemisphere. Complete surgical removal is feasible.

In most children presentation is with unilateral ataxia, as the tumour commonly arises from one or other hemisphere; and ultimately with the signs of raised ICP. The peak incidence appears to be between the ages of five and 10 years.

The diagnosis, as with medulloblastoma, depends upon the history, clinical examination, skull x-rays, CAT scan, and surgical exploration of the posterior fossa.

Treatment is largely surgical as the role or advantages of radiotherapy are controversial. Survival may be prolonged even if total surgical removal is not possible.

Ependymoma

An ependymoma is a tumour that arises from the ependymal lining of the ventricular system of the brain. While most ependymomas in children arise in the posterior fossa from the floor of the fourth ventricle, a few may arise from the brain above the tentorium. Ependymomas are slightly more common in males and tend to occur early in childhood.

Posterior fossa ependymomas often present with raised ICP but because the growth originates in the floor of the fourth ventricle some cranial nerve signs may be evident and be part of the initial clinical presentation. Furthermore, the tumour may extend laterally and occupy what is known as the cerebello-pontine angle, where involvement of the sixth nerve (producing a squint), the seventh nerve (producing facial weakness), and the eighth nerve (causing deafness and unsteadiness) will be clinically apparent.

Diagnosis may be suggested from the clinical picture and radiological studies but as with most posterior fossa tumours surgical exploration is necessary for diagnostic confirmation.

Ependymomas cannot be totally removed. Undue manipulation at surgery may compromise the vital centres that exist in the floor of the fourth ventricle, so affecting blood pressure, heart rate, and respiratory function.

Radiotherapy is indicated after surgery, although the outlook is poor and the survival far less than that for medulloblastomas.

Brainstem gliomas

These occur most commonly in the pons and present at a mean age of seven years with multiple cranial nerve palsies and commonly some dysfunction of the long descending (pyramidal) tracts. Cranial nerves will be involved on both sides of the midline. A raised ICP tends to be a late sign.

Plain skull x-rays may be normal but a CAT scan will demonstrate the swelling of the brainstem. Radiological signs taken together with the clinical picture will provide the diagnosis. A biopsy may sometimes be attempted but this is often technically difficult.

While treatment with radiotherapy is advocated and may well be responsible for increasing the survival time for most children, the overall outlook remains very poor. Survival for more than a few months is unusual.

Gliomas of the optic pathways and hypothalamus

The eye and optic tracts are part of the brain and because they are composed of glial tissue may develop glial tumours. Many of these tumours are associated with von Recklinghausen's disease (see Chapter 16) and can be associated with prolonged survival due to the very slow tumour growth rate.

The clinical presentation will depend largely upon where in the optic pathway the tumour arises. If the tumour is within the orbit the commonest sign will be that of protrusion of the eye (proptosis) but with normal eye movement. Vision may be only mildly impaired and swelling of the optic nerve head (papilloedema) may be seen although atrophy of the optic disc is more common.

If the tumour is in the head (intracranial) it will commonly cause visual loss and very often optic nerve atrophy because of pressure or invasion. At the time of diagnosis these signs and symptoms are usually extensive and it is often difficult to decide the exact position of the lesion.

If a tumour involves the hypothalamus then growth may be adversely affected because of endocrine abnormalities. If an obstruction of CSF circulation to the third ventricle occurs because of tumour size this may result in hydrocephalus with raised ICP.

Appropriate x-rays of the skull may show the signs of raised ICP, erosion of the foramina in the orbit through which the optic nerves pass, and erosion of the anterior clinoid processes of the pituitary fossa to form the so-called 'J-shaped fossa'. CAT scans further define the position and extent of the tumour.

The slow growth of these tumours has rendered the arguments

over definitive treatment complex. In the presence of a definite optic nerve tumour some have argued that resection of the nerve with or without enucleation of the eye should be performed. Others have argued that the treatment be confined solely to radiotherapy, and yet a third group suggest no treatment at all. In the cases of the second and third lines of approach *very* careful follow-up is obviously indicated.

Craniopharyngioma

This is the commonest brain tumour in childhood that is not of glial origin and is one of several varieties of tumours situated above the pituitary fossa (suprasellar).

It apparently originates from an embryonic remnant —Rathke's pouch. The tumour may sometimes be within the pituitary fossa, although in most cases it is above. The tumour itself is usually at least partially cystic, often containing calcium within the cyst wall.

The presentation of such tumours may be with raised ICP due to the size of the tumour or its obstruction to CSF flow, visual disturbance due to pressure on the optic chiasm or some disturbance of the pituitary gland. This last problem may result in diabetes insipidus (a failure of the kidney to concentrate urine due to the absence of antidiuretic hormone, a hormone excreted by the posterior part of the pituitary gland), growth failure (due to the absence of the secretion of growth hormone from the anterior pituitary gland) as well as bouts of stupor, fever, hypoglycaemia and hypotension resulting from interference with hypothalamic function.

Definitive diagnosis can be aided by plain skull radiography which may show the calcium within the tumour and distortion of the pituitary fossa, and a CAT scan will usually demonstrate the tumour clearly. Endocrinological tests often suggest pituitary dysfunction.

The principal aim of surgical treatment is to decompress the tumour by aspirating the cystic portions. Fortunately, most craniopharyngiomas are relatively benign but total removal is usually impossible because of adherence to vital structures. Radiotherapy may be used in addition to surgery to help prevent recurrence. Together with this the treatment of associated hydrocephalus with a shunt may be necessary and endocrine replacement therapy will almost always be needed.

The outlook in children with craniopharyngiomas is generally favourable, although relapse due to an increase in the size of the tumour may occur and thus surgical re-exploration may be required.

It would appear that brain tumours in childhood are generally diagnosed late from a failure to recognise that the headache, vomiting, and listlessness are not due to a viral infection or gastroenteritis but raised ICP. Whether earlier diagnosis might improve the results of treatment has to remain speculative.

FURTHER READING

Bell, W. E. and McCormich, W. F. (1978). *Increased Intracranial Pressure in Children*, 2nd edition. W. B. Saunders Co, Philadelphia.

Matson, D. D. (1969). *Neurosurgery of Infancy and Childhood*, 2nd edition. Charles C. Thomas, Springfield, Illinois.

Till, K. (1975). *Paediatric Neurosurgery for Paediatricians and Neurosurgeons*. Blackwell Scientific Publications Limited, Oxford.

COMMON NEUROLOGICAL
SYMPTOMS

13. The floppy baby

All young babies are, to a degree, floppy and the newborn infant has minimal head control. The premature baby often exhibits an increased amount of floppiness or hypotonia. The term *floppy infant syndrome* is reserved for a group of infants whose floppiness or hypotonia is inappropriate for their age or stage of development. In whatever position the infant with severe floppiness is placed or held—pull to sit, ventrosuspension, prone, or supine—the appearances closely resemble that of a rag doll (Fig. 13/1). When laid supine the infant will adopt a position reminiscent of a frog. Many infants who are floppy are also weak; depending on the severity of this there may be varying degrees of reduction in the movements of the limbs, poor respiratory

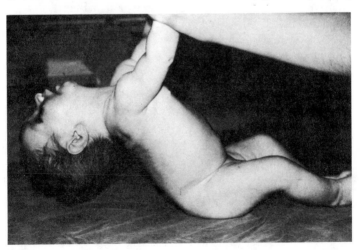

Fig. 13/1 The 'floppy baby'

movements, a weak cry, and poor sucking. In addition the floppy infant 'feels' different to a normal baby when held. The floppy infant syndrome is not a diagnosis but a description. In these babies it is a matter of some urgency for a cause of the floppiness to be sought.

Generally, the diagnostic possibilities may be divided into three major groups.

GENERAL DISORDERS

Prematurity has already been mentioned as a cause of floppiness. In addition any unwell neonate or infant will often be, apart from apathetic, floppy. Severe infection, electrolyte imbalance, congenital heart disease, gastro-intestinal disease, renal disease, some metabolic disorders, or hypothermia may produce a young child who is weak, apathetic, and floppy.

CENTRAL NERVOUS SYSTEM DISORDERS

Many infants who have sustained some perinatal insult may, at least initially, be floppy as well as possibly irritable. Tendon reflexes in these infants may be very brisk and the patterns of movement may be abnormal.

Children with Down's syndrome are extremely floppy at birth.

NEUROMUSCULAR DISORDERS

These disorders produce floppiness associated with weakness due to disease or dysfunction of the *motor unit*. The motor unit is accepted as including the whole nerve from the spinal cord to the nerve ending and the muscle it supplies (the nucleus of a motor nerve situated at the anterior horn of the spinal column, the nerve trunk, the neuromuscular junction, and the muscle itself).

Diseases of the motor unit may be divided into two major groups. Firstly, neuropathic disease such as spinal muscular atrophy and congenital neuropathies where the principal defect is in the nerve or its nucleus in the anterior horn of the spinal cord. Secondly, myopathic diseases including the congenital myopathies and dystrophia myotonica, where the muscle itself is primarily affected.

Neuromuscular investigations

Before considering the diseases that come under these groupings it might be fitting to consider some of the investigations that are commonly used in a child suspected of a neuromuscular disorder.

CREATINE PHOSPHOKINASE (CPK)

This enzyme is present in high levels within the skeletal muscle and some other tissues. When a muscle is damaged for whatever reason, there will be a leakage of CPK into the bloodstream and the levels in the blood will be higher than usual. The highest levels are normally found in myopathic lesions, particularly in the Duchenne type of muscular dystrophy (see Chapter 14). Some elevation is often seen in the neuropathic lesions but normal levels are common and the elevations when they occur, are not striking.

ELECTROMYOGRAPHY (EMG)

This is the electrophysiological study of the motor unit. The EMG has direct parallels with both the EEG and the ECG. With EMG studies the electrical activity of an active muscle is identified and displayed on an oscilloscope. The electrical patterns of the muscle potentials of normal children are known and deviations can be suggestive either of a neuropathic or a myopathic disorder. The integrity and normality of peripheral nerves can be studied by electrical stimulation and measurement of the speed of conduction of an impulse along the nerves. Various neuropathies can be diagnosed with this technique.

MUSCLE BIOPSY

This is often diagnostically useful. A sample is usually obtained from a large proximal muscle group using either a small operative technique or a muscle biopsy needle. This enables the study of the structure of the muscle to be made with special staining techniques.

SPINAL MUSCULAR ATROPHIES

There are several different types of spinal muscular atrophy but in all of these the fundamental defect is damage to, or loss of, the nuclei of the motor nerves in the anterior horn of the spinal cord.

Werdnig-Hoffmann disease

The most well known and severe form of spinal muscular atrophy is Werdnig-Hoffmann disease. Affected infants are usually extremely weak at birth, and there may be a history of decreased fetal movement. A small proportion of infants may be born relatively physically normal but with severe weakness developing within the first few weeks of life.

Not only is there marked weakness in affected infants but also severe respiratory difficulty and a bell-shaped chest because of intercostal muscle weakness. Additionally there may be sufficient weakness, particularly in the bulbar muscles, to produce swallowing and sucking difficulties. Possible immobility during fetal life is responsible for a large number of joint contractures present in children with Werdnig-Hoffmann disease. Muscle bulk is reduced. The tongue may have a peculiar trembling appearance due to miniature contractions of muscles. This is known as muscle fasciculation. Usually the face is unaffected by muscle weakness and the infants may have a very 'wide awake' appearance. Tendon reflexes are absent.

The CPK is frequently elevated although not markedly and may even be normal. The EMG examination demonstrates loss of functioning nerves. Studies of the peripheral nerves may show mild reduction in the velocity of conduction but the findings in this part of the study are largely normal. If a biopsy is performed very small muscle fibres will be seen throughout the biopsy sample.

The outlook with Werdnig-Hoffmann disease is always very poor. Survival past the first year of life is unusual and past the second, rare. This is due to a combination of factors; firstly, the weakness is so profound that chest infections invariably occur and are difficult to treat, and secondly the condition is not entirely static and may be associated with increasing weakness.

Werdnig-Hoffmann disease is genetically determined and is autosomally recessively inherited. This means that the parents of an affected child have a one in four chance of subsequently having a similarly affected infant.

Intermediate form spinal muscular atrophy

This form of spinal muscular atrophy is sometimes referred to as SMA type II, with Werdnig-Hoffmann disease referred to as SMA type I.

With this form of spinal muscular atrophy infants are nearly always normal in their early motor milestones, and the ability to sit may be at the usual age of between five and six months. After this there appears to be very little motor progress; weakness is often quite marked, being more obvious in the legs than the arms. Respiratory and bulbar muscles are less commonly affected than in Werdnig-Hoffmann disease. The face is usually spared. The trembling fasciculation of the tongue is more commonly seen in the intermediate form of spinal muscular atrophy. There may be a coarse tremor of the outstretched hand. The cause of the tremor and muscle fasciculation is thought to be due to the surviving anterior horn cell nuclei attempting to re-innervate muscle, not in an orderly fashion but randomly so that there is little control over small nerve fibres activating equally small muscle fibres.

Creatine phosphokinase levels are usually normal but the EMG examination reveals a fairly typical picture that points to a loss of active nerve fibres but also identifies the attempted reinnervation of the muscle.

The muscle biopsy sample is characterised by groups of very small fibres immediately adjacent to groups of very large fibres.

Contractures around joints occur and the development of scoliosis is a particular hazard. For their survival these children require active treatment to prevent contractures and particularly to prevent scoliosis. Judicious bracing combined at times with surgical orthopaedic procedures may allow some form of ambulation for a small proportion of children. The outlook generally will depend upon the degree of respiratory involvement and the progression of the disorder. In some children, once the clinical picture has developed, continuing progressive weakness does not occur.

The genetic pattern is the same as Werdnig-Hoffmann disease. In both these conditions there is no method at present for antenatal diagnosis.

CONGENITAL NEUROPATHIES

Neuropathies are uncommon in infants but do occur and may be difficult to distinguish from other neuropathic and myopathic conditions on clinical grounds alone. Measurement of nerve conduction velocities are helpful in diagnosis. In most, no known cause exists for congenital neuropathies, although very occasionally they are linked with some rare neurodegenerative disorder.

CONGENITAL MYOPATHIES

Because of the availability of newer and more specialised means of studying muscle biopsy samples, a large number of congenital myopathies have now been identified. Those described in this chapter are the best known. They are differentiated from each other principally by the appearance of the biopsy. With a greater application of these modern techniques the clinical picture associated with the different forms of myopathy is beginning to emerge.

Creatine phosphokinase estimations are often normal and the EMG will also either be normal or may show a typically myopathic picture. As a group most of these patients have definite but not necessarily severe weakness with hypotonia and delayed motor milestones. Progression of the disease, although it often occurs, is not invariable.

Central core disease

This is a congenital myopathy in which the muscle fibres will show holes or cores on biopsy examination.

The outlook for these children is generally good, although they may show a slight deterioration in later childhood. It is important that care is taken to prevent secondary joint contractures and that respiratory infections are adequately treated.

The condition is autosomally dominantly inherited, which means that parents with one affected child stand a 50 per cent chance of having another who is similarly affected. Furthermore some parents, although healthy, may on biopsy be shown to have the characteristic findings of this disorder.

Nemaline myopathy (rod-body myopathy)

This condition, like other congenital myopathies, will be characterised generally by floppiness, weakness and delayed motor milestones, together with poor muscle bulk. Many such children will have a long, thin face and high palate. Scoliosis is more common than in other congenital myopathies. Pes cavus (high arches to the feet) is sometimes seen in later childhood. The specific diagnosis is made from the biopsy samples, which on appropriate staining will show rod-like bodies in the muscle fibres.

Affected children may sometimes show mild progressive deterioration and death has been reported from respiratory insufficiency late in childhood or early adult life.

Genetically, nemaline myopathy may occur sporadically; but as with central core disease, it may be an autosomal dominantly inherited condition.

Myotubular myopathy (central nuclear myopathy)

As well as generalised floppiness many patients with this myopathy will have droopy eyes (ptosis) and some restriction of eye movements, with facial and truncal weakness.

The biopsy appearances are similar to those seen in early fetal life with a high proportion of the nuclei of the muscle fibres being in the centre of the fibre rather than at the edge. Walking normally starts by the age of two years. The progression of muscle weakness is variable. For some patients a static course is seen while in others there is a mild deterioration and the development of various skeletal abnormalities such as scoliosis and pes cavus.

The genetic pattern is variable. Myotubular myopathy has been reported in more than one member of a family and again, as in the case of central core disease, apparently clinically unaffected relatives may have the biopsy appearances associated with this condition. Overall it seems more likely that the condition is autosomally dominantly inherited.

Congenital muscular dystrophy

Congenital muscular dystrophy is a congenital myopathy perhaps worthy of special mention, because of the confusion its name can sometimes cause. The confusion arises because it is assumed to be the same as the muscular dystrophy seen in boys at a later age which is associated with severe progressive weakness. Congenital muscular dystrophy is, however, probably more than one condition. Gross distortion of the normal muscle architecture, similar to that seen in other forms of dystrophy, is noted on biopsy. Some affected children will slowly improve with time, others will remain static, and others will show a definite downhill course. Joint contractures may be severe, present at birth, and be reminiscent of a so-called 'arthrogryposis syndrome'. Physiotherapy and orthopaedic surgery are important.

The general pattern of inheritance is autosomally recessive.

Dystrophia myotonica

This condition is well recognised in adults, although rare. Only recently has the existence of a congenital form of this condition been recognised.

Dystrophia myotonica is characterised by muscle weakness and wasting in some muscles more than others and *myotonia*—the inability of a muscle, once it has contracted, to relax readily. This may mean that on shaking hands the affected individual has difficulty in relaxing the grip.

The mother of a child with congenital dystrophia myotonica usually has the condition herself, although it may never have been diagnosed. Such mothers often have long, thin faces and when asked to tightly close the eyes are unable to do so because of slight facial muscle weakness. Also, when they are asked to squeeze a finger or similar object they have difficulty in relaxing their grip. Affected pregnancies may often be characterised by excess liquor (hydramnios). Marked respiratory difficulties, a poor suck, and profound floppiness are common in the neonatal period and early infancy. Postural abnormalities of the feet may be present at birth. The neonatal difficulties are sufficiently severe to cause death in some affected children. In survivors the respiratory and feeding difficulties improve in a relatively short time. The facial appearance of the affected individuals is characteristic. The mouth is open, droopy, and 'fish-like'.

Developmental progress is often somewhat slow and mental retardation is common. The variety of diagnostic tests referred to previously will, in infancy, give entirely normal results and the diagnosis is made from both the child's general appearance and detecting the condition in the mother.

Congenital dystrophia myotonica is dominantly inherited and careful studies of the families of affected children suggest that several members have the disorder subclinically. It is clearly important for careful genetic advice to be given to the whole family, especially the female members. It is suspected that part of the aetiology of the congenital form of dystrophia myotonica is due to a so-called 'maternal factor' that crosses the placenta and causes the severe neonatal difficulties.

PRADER-WILLI SYNDROME
(HYPOTONIA—OBESITY SYNDROME)

Although affected infants are markedly floppy at birth, there is nothing definite to suggest that this disorder is primarily neuromuscular. As well as the severe floppiness, there is accompanying early feeding difficulty and a weak cry. The head is usually disproportionately large and the face has a characteristic appearance with the eyes being rather almond shaped, the hair initially fair, and the eyes blue. In the male the testes are either very small or absent and the scrotum is rudimentary.

With age floppiness and feeding difficulties resolve and reasonable motor progress is accomplished. An insatiable appetite is common in the second or third year of life and if this is not controlled obesity results. Mental retardation is invariable.

Investigations for a neuromuscular disorder are usually normal. The bone age may be retarded. The diagnosis is made on clinical grounds.

One of the major problems in the management of these children is the control of their diet and the prevention of overeating. Children with Prader-Willi syndrome are short and may develop diabetes at a later age.

The disorder is not thought to be genetically determined but some chromosome abnormalities have been described.

In the past a floppy infant received various so-called diagnostic labels. These included benign congenital hypotonia or amyotonia congenita. It is now realised that such labels are artificial and that every floppy infant requires a disciplined diagnostic approach so that a specific diagnosis can be made, affording an opportunity towards prognostications, a rational approach towards what treatment is available and, most important, fair and reliable genetic advice to the parents of such children.

FURTHER READING

Dubowitz, V. (1969). *The Floppy Infant Syndrome*. Spastics International Medical Publications. Clinics in Developmental Medicine, No 31. William Heinemann Medical Books Ltd, London.

Dubowitz, V. (1978). *Muscle Disorders in Childhood*. W. B. Saunders Co, Philadelphia.

Walton, J. N. (Ed) (1974). *Disorders of Voluntary Muscle*, 3rd edition. Churchill Livingstone, Edinburgh.

14. Progressive muscle weakness

A group of diseases are described in this chapter which present as progressive muscle weakness during childhood. These are neuromuscular diseases which, unlike the congenital neuromuscular diseases described in Chapter 13 are preceded by normal development. The common presenting sign is that of locomotor difficulty. This results from lower limb weakness, which usually causes problems before that of the upper limbs.

These diseases can be divided into two major groups—those that affect the muscle itself, as in the muscular dystrophies, and those that affect the nervous system, as in the hereditary neuropathies.

MUSCULAR DYSTROPHY

The word dystrophy implies an actively destructive disorder. There are several differing types of muscular dystrophy of which the most common and severe form is that described by Duchenne and often referred to as pseudohypertrophic muscular dystrophy. The prevalence is approximately three per 100 000 or between 13 and 33 per 100 000 liveborn males.

Duchenne muscular dystrophy

This condition is X-linked recessive and therefore occurs only in boys. In two-thirds of cases the mother will be a carrier, although without symptoms; in one-third of these there will be a family history that makes it obvious that the mother must be a carrier. In the remaining one-third there is no certain method of assessing carrier status, but a very high probability estimate can be made using blood CPK (see p. 169) estimations. The genetic question must be examined as soon as the diagnosis is made, to reduce the risk of further affected individuals being born, but because of the often late diagnosis of the condition, other affected siblings may already be born. At present there is considerable discussion about the feasibility and desirability of neonatal screening of all male infants, or alternatively the screening of all males who are not walking by the age of 18 months. There is, however, the difficult question as to whether one should diagnose conditions before they become clinically apparent when there is no definitive treatment available.

The diagnosis of Duchenne muscular dystrophy is commonly made between the ages of three and five years, although parents may well have been aware of significant abnormalities in neuromuscular function long before that time. Often they have been reassured that the child is 'lazy', 'flat-footed', or 'clumsy'.

The presenting complaints are problems with walking and running—particularly on going up slopes or stairs—a waddling gait due to pelvic girdle weakness, frequent falling, and difficulty getting up from the floor or low chairs. In the early stages difficulties with the arms are relatively uncommon, but later there are comments about the inability to raise hands above the head and with specific tasks like combing the hair.

Observation of boys getting up from the floor will reveal the characteristic manoeuvre known as *Gowers' sign* (Fig. 14/1). Because of the pelvic girdle weakness the boy has to roll onto his front and then push against his thighs to straighten up. This is described as 'climbing up oneself'. There is wasting in several muscle groups; on the other hand some muscles appear to be hypertrophied (bulky), particularly those of the calf and sometimes the deltoid and other shoulder muscles.

It is known that up to a third of boys with Duchenne muscular dystrophy have some degree of learning difficulty or mental retardation and at times this mental retardation is of such significance that the co-existent neuromuscular dysfunction is overlooked—at least in early childhood.

Investigations commonly performed in the evaluation of

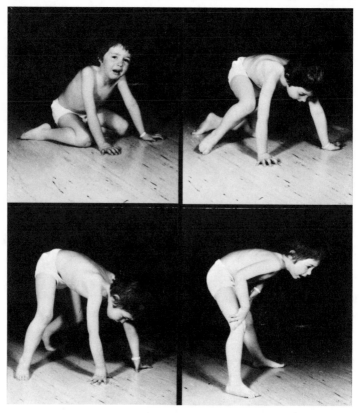

Fig. 14/1 Gowers' sign

neuromuscular disorders have already been described in Chapter 13.

Measurement of blood CPK in Duchenne dystrophy reveals exceedingly high levels of this enzyme in the circulation. An EMG examination will demonstrate markedly myopathic potentials and a biopsy of the muscle will demonstrate gross distortion of the normal structure with infiltration by fat and fibrous tissue (Figs 14/2 and 14/3). It is this infiltration that produces the bulky

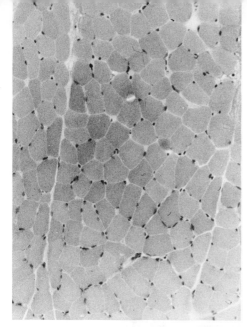

Fig. 14/2
A normal muscle
biopsy

Fig. 14/3
Muscle biopsy in early
Duchenne dystropy

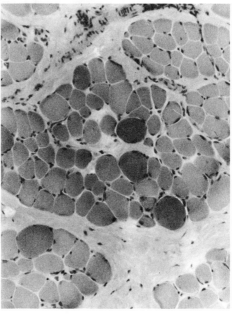

appearance in some of the muscles and is the origin of the term 'pseudohypertrophy'.

Cardiac muscle is affected as well as skeletal muscle and this can be reflected in abnormalities seen on the ECG in some boys with Duchenne type muscular dystrophy.

The course of this illness is one of steady deterioration in locomotor function, although a static phase may be seen in the early years after the diagnosis is made. Virtually all the boys are off their feet and in a wheelchair by the age of 12 years. While the initial presentation is difficulty in walking, at a later age arm weakness becomes very apparent. This means that not only is a wheelchair required for mobility but it has to be electrically powered (Fig. 14/4).

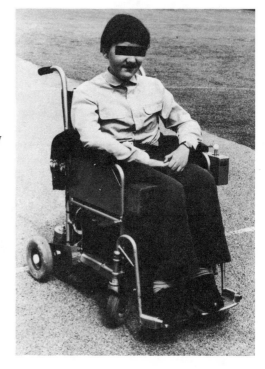

Fig. 14/4
Teenage boy with
Duchenne dystrophy
using an electric
wheelchair

Duchenne dystrophy poses very significant stress not only on the parents but also on those that come into contact with the child professionally. Each boy and his family must be treated as an individual and this particularly applies not only at the time of diagnosis but also at a later stage when ambulation is no longer possible. Much work has been undertaken on the use of long leg splints to prolong the time a boy may be able to walk and various orthopaedic procedures have, in some cases, proved to be helpful. Clinical experience suggests that by the time most boys acquire a wheelchair they are very ready and glad to receive it, although the parents may feel differently.

During the ambulatory phase a moderate amount of exercise is advisable together with attention paid to preventing contractures of the hips and ankles by regularly instituted passive stretching. The use of night splints is controversial. Perhaps as important as anything is the avoidance of undue immobilisation. This is important not only in Duchenne dystrophy but also in other neuromuscular disorders where it is recognised that a period of immobilisation may have a detrimental effect on subsequent locomotor function. A child with a muscular dystrophy who has to undergo surgery or who has an infective illness must be mobilised as soon as possible. The prevention of obesity, which can be difficult, is even more important.

When a wheelchair becomes inevitable, care must be taken that the chair prescribed is appropriate to the individual boy. Chairs should have a sloping back which helps to prevent scoliosis—a major complication of muscular dystrophy. Adequate support for the feet is important to prevent contractures at the ankles and the development of talipes equinovarus, which causes not only discomfort but also difficulties with shoe fitting. Most important of all, it must be appreciated that the chair has to be functional not only for mobility but also for a variety of daily tasks, including school work.

Because the natural course of this disorder is towards a progressive weakening of all skeletal muscles, the risks of respiratory infections are high. Death may well occur any time from the teens to the early twenties as the result of either respiratory disease or cardiomyopathy.

Becker dystrophy

This condition, like Duchenne dystrophy, is X linked and in some ways may be considered similar. The severity of this muscular dystrophy is much less and the presentation will be at a later age, with most patients affected being ambulant until at least into early adult life. Ultimately the weakness becomes sufficiently severe to require a wheelchair.

Diagnosis depends upon detection of high levels of CPK in the blood, the finding of a myopathic EMG, and a biopsy in which the appearances of the muscle may be similar to that of Duchenne type dystrophy.

Here again, there are female carriers of this form of dystrophy who may be identified by blood CPK estimations.

Limb girdle dystrophy

There are two principal forms of this type of muscular dystrophy. A pelvi-femoral type exists in which the pelvic girdle is predominantly affected and a facio-scapulo-humeral form in which a number of muscles in the shoulder girdle are affected and there is an associated facial weakness.

The first form of limb girdle dystrophy is very much more common than the second and clinically it is difficult to distinguish from Becker dystrophy when it occurs in boys. Indeed with CPK and EMG examinations there may be similarities and even on muscle biopsy it can still be difficult to differentiate one from the other. The age of onset can be extremely variable but commonly it is towards the end of the first decade of life or in the teens.

The genetic pattern is usually autosomally recessive. This means that the parents of an affected child may have a one in four chance of producing another similarly affected child.

The progression of this disorder is variable. As with Becker dystrophy, the tendency is towards a variable but slow deterioration of locomotor function. This results in the need for a wheelchair at least towards the end of young adult life.

In the facio-scapulo-humeral dystrophy the onset is normally that of weakness in the muscles of the face and shoulders; this weakness ultimately spreads to the proximal muscles of the lower limbs. The age of presentation is usually the teens or early twenties. Progression is slow.

The genetic pattern in this condition is complicated because examination of the families of affected individuals may reveal minimal signs of the condition. It is possibly an example of dominant inheritance so that the parents of an affected child have a 50 per cent chance of producing a similarly affected child. On the other hand, sporadic occurrence would seem to be common.

KUGELBERG-WELANDER'S DISEASE

This is a form of spinal muscular atrophy and is related to Werdnig-Hoffmann disease (SMA type I) and intermediate-form spinal muscular atrophy (SMA type II). (For further details see Chapter 13.) Although the defect is in the anterior horn cells in the spinal cord the clinical picture is totally different from the most severe infantile forms of spinal muscular atrophy.

The presenting symptoms are similar to those of a limb girdle dystrophy. Tendon reflexes are depressed or absent and fasciculation or 'rippling' of muscle is readily seen.

Apart from clinical clues there are a number of factors which are diagnostically useful. The levels of CPK are near to, or within, the normal range and the EMG will suggest a neuropathic rather than a myopathic condition. The diagnosis may ultimately depend upon a muscle biopsy showing a number of small atrophic fibres closely associated with groups of massively enlarged or hypertrophic fibres.

The outlook for the future in such children is variable. In many there may be little progression over many years, although ultimately there is deterioration in locomotor function. In others there will be a steady progressive deterioration of function with significant neuromuscular difficulties in middle adult life.

Kugelberg-Welander's disease is autosomally recessively inherited.

DERMATOMYOSITIS

A mild non-specific illness may precede the onset of muscle pain and weakness that are the characteristic symptoms of dermatomyositis. Together with this a number of skin changes are described. A purple rash may be found over the face, knuckles, elbows, and knees. Weakness is principally of proximal muscles and early muscle wasting is prominent; the neck flexor muscles are markedly involved in the early stages of the disease.

The CPK level may be normal or extremely high and the EMG examination may show marked myopathic potentials, or be normal. Commonly a biopsy will show evidence of inflammatory changes within the muscle associated with atrophy of fibres, particularly in those near to blood vessels.

As soon as possible after the onset of the illness dermatomyositis is treated with high doses of steroids. Response to therapy is usually gratifying but it may be necessary to use steroids or other anti-inflammatory agents over prolonged periods of time. Care is needed to administer the minimal dose compatible with the patient's reasonable muscle function.

NEUROPATHIES

Neuropathies produce weakness and wasting of the more distal muscles, together with absent reflexes and often pes cavus. A flapping, stamping gait, together with a clawing of the toes due to weakness of the intrinsic foot muscles is more common than the waddling gait seen with disorders of muscle. Sensory impairment may be present.

Neuropathies in childhood may be seen associated with more widespread disease of the central nervous system and with some metabolic disorders. Drugs such as the antineoplastic agent vincristine may cause neuropathies. There is a large group of familial or hereditary neuropathies.

Charcot-Marie-Tooth disease

This is also known as peroneal muscular atrophy because of the early involvement of the peroneal group of muscles as well as the small intrinsic muscles of the feet. The early signs of Charcot-Marie-Tooth disease are usually in the feet. Development of pes cavus and clawing of the toes is secondary to the weakness of the small muscles of the feet, producing difficulty in walking and shoe fitting and often associated with pain. The rate of progression of weakness and the involvement of other below-knee muscles is variable. Atrophy and loss of muscle bulk is common in the affected muscles. Hand and wrist muscles are commonly affected at a later stage of the illness. Loss of peripheral sensation occurs but is not invariable.

The diagnosis is usually relatively straightforward on clinical grounds alone. Care has to be taken to distinguish Charcot-Marie-Tooth disease from a neuropathy secondary to one of the more generalised metabolic or degenerative conditions. In a high proportion of cases nerve conduction studies demonstrate marked slowing of transmission along the nerves. In some cases of Charcot-Marie-Tooth disease biopsy of the nerve may reveal a loss of the myelin layer and 'onion bulbing' due to marked thickening in various segments of the nerves. In other cases of Charcot-Marie-Tooth disease, the biopsy suggests that the axon of the nerve is most at fault, and the surrounding myelin layer is reasonably normal. In this latter group measurements of nerve conduction will often be normal.

The disease progression is very variable, but for the majority of patients it is slow, and ambulation can be expected for prolonged periods of time. The early involvement of orthopaedic surgeons in the management of this condition is important as much can be done surgically both to alleviate the discomfort in the feet and to produce as efficient walking as possible.

Guillain-Barré syndrome (infectious polyneuritis)

Occasionally, a short time after a viral infection there may be a rapid onset of generalised weakness resulting from inflammation of nerves. The presentation of this disorder may well be with paraesthesia in the feet and hands, together with severe pain in the legs due to inflammation of sensory nerves. Weakness is initially most marked in the legs and may spread upwards to involve not only arms but also the respiratory muscles. Rapid progression may occur for one or two weeks followed by a static phase before a very slow improvement takes place over a prolonged period of time.

Examination of the cerebrospinal fluid shows a high level of protein but no inflammatory cells. This finding may not be present at the onset of the illness but in many cases occurs later, perhaps during recovery.

Guillain-Barré syndrome can be a very severe illness and patients may need to be nursed in an intensive care unit so that support can be given if the respiratory muscles become affected. Attention to other factors such as the risks of hypotension and cardiac arrhythmias is important.

Steroids are given to some patients, although there is no evidence that they have any beneficial effect in the treatment of this condition.

MYASTHENIA GRAVIS

In this disorder the progressive fatiguing of muscles is the principal feature. In the commonest form it has now been demonstrated that the receptors of the nerve transmitter *acetyl choline*, which are at the neuromuscular junction, are predominantly 'blocked' by an immunoglobulin. Abnormalities are noted in the thymus gland in over 75 per cent of children and young adults with myasthenia gravis.

Weakness of muscle is characteristically increased by exercise but, unlike normal fatigue, pain is not a feature.

The eyelids are involved in virtually all patients, causing them to droop (ptosis); many patients will have limb weakness—proximal and distal weakness; weakness of the bulbar muscles; and facial weakness, with swallowing and speech difficulties. Respiratory difficulties may occur in those most severely affected. Patients can be grouped according to their clinical severity—some only having ocular problems while others have severe respiratory difficulties. Those only mildly affected will show fatigue and weakness only with moderate exercise. This weakness may be reversed for a short time by giving edrophonium chloride (Tensilon) by injection. Repetitive stimulation of a nerve may, on EMG examination, demonstrate decrement of the muscle action potential.

In children myasthenia gravis may be split into three groups.

NEONATAL MYASTHENIA

This is a transitory disorder lasting less than a month that occurs in about 10 per cent of the babies of mothers with myasthenia gravis.

CONGENITAL MYASTHENIA GRAVIS

This is very rare, and presents shortly after birth or at least in very early infancy. It does not tend to get worse, and there is no evidence of immunoglobulin blocking of the receptors at the neuromuscular junction.

JUVENILE MYASTHENIA

This the commonest form of myasthenia that can present during childhood or young adulthood; the clinical features have been described above.

Treatment

The main form of therapy is the giving of anticholinesterase drugs—pyridostigmine and the shorter-acting neostigmine. Dosage and timing have to be very carefully arranged so as to exert the maximum effect for the whole day without causing side-effects. In addition steroids given on alternate days may be needed in some more severely affected patients.

Thymectomy (the removal of the thymus gland) is beneficial to many patients with juvenile myasthenia gravis (but not with congenital myasthenia) and long remissions may be expected.

With careful management and medication the majority of children with myasthenia gravis are able to live normal or near normal lives.

Many of the neuromuscular disorders in children have no specific therapy. This does not mean that there are no good reasons to strive for a specific diagnosis; there are both prognostic and genetic reasons. As well as this, besides the majority of neuromuscular disorders which are 'untreatable' there are a few that do have a specific treatment.

While admitting that many of the conditions are without specific treatment this does not mean that there is nothing for the nurse, therapist, or doctor to do once a firm diagnosis has been made. There are many aspects of management such as the prevention of joint contractures, scoliosis, and obesity which are vitally important in preserving the maximum neuromuscular function for as long as possible. Apart from this a caring, supportive relationship towards the patient and the family is of obvious importance.

FURTHER READING

Dubowitz, V. and Brooke, M. H. (1973). *Muscle Biopsy: A Modern Approach*. W. B. Saunders Co, Philadelphia.

Dubowitz, V. (1978). *Muscle Disorders in Childhood*. W. B. Saunders Co, Philadelphia.

Walton, J. N. (Ed) (1974). *Disorders of Voluntary Muscle*, 3rd edition. Churchill Livingstone, Edinburgh.

15. Ataxia: co-ordination difficulties

Ataxia is a feature most commonly associated with a disorder of the cerebellum or the cerebellar connections. It results from defective control and irregularity of voluntary muscle movement.

The cerebellum is that part of the brain associated with control of the rate, range, direction, and force of voluntary movement.

It is important to consider other causes of inco-ordination which might be confused with cerebellar ataxia. Inco-ordination may be caused by proprioceptive disorders (the orientation of the body in space—position sense); the presence of muscle weakness; sensory abnormalities; and conditions, such as chorea and myoclonus, in which there are uncontrolled added muscle movement. Conditions producing muscle weakness and those associated with uncontrolled added movement have been discussed previously.

This chapter will concentrate on ataxia itself and the conditions in which this seems to be the principal defect or disorder. It will consider disorders of the cerebellum, its connections, and some other causes of ataxia.

In cerebellar disease, arm function may be disturbed by a tremor which is more marked when movements are attempted—an intention tremor. This may be seen when attempting to reach for and grasp objects. The tremor will become more marked the nearer the hand is to the object. Fine manipulative movements necessary for doing up and undoing buttons will be impaired. The formal finger-nose-finger testing in the neurological examination is a means of identifying this type of dysfunction. The ability to manipulate small pegs into a pegboard may identify difficulties in manipulative function and rapid hand movements may reveal difficulties. If the outstretched hands are tapped when the eyes are closed there will be a marked 'overshoot' in returning to the original position in the presence of cerebellar dysfunction.

Ataxia of the trunk (truncal ataxia), with midline cerebellar disorders, renders sitting without support difficult.

Abnormalities of eye movement with cerebellar dysfunction are common. Nystagmus reflects a disturbance of the balance of fixation of the eyes resulting in a drift in one or other direction with a quick compensatory movement back to the midline. When this cycle is continually repeated nystagmus is said to exist. The most common nystagmus is horizontal, but there may also be forms with a rotary component in disorders at the level of the foramen magnum and a vertical nystagmus when there is involvement of the cerebellar tonsils.

With midline cerebellar disorders speech may be jerky, explosive, and slurred—dysarthric. An abnormality of a cerebellar hemisphere may give rise to difficulty in walking, with a staggering gait towards the affected side (ataxic gait) and other signs suggesting poor cerebellar function on that side of the body. In cerebellar disease the gait will almost certainly be wide-based and staggering.

Non-cerebellar causes of ataxia

Acute ataxia may be due to the ingestion of toxic substances or drugs. The anticonvulsants phenytoin (Epanutin), primidone (Mysoline) and phenobarbitone (Luminal) are known causes of such problems. Alcohol must not be forgotten!

ACUTE CEREBELLAR ATAXIA

Acute viral cerebellitis

Encephalitides (see Chapter 10) may occasionally affect primarily the cerebellum and be accompanied by other signs of an encephalitic illness, e.g. fever, headaches, lethargy, and irritability. Changes in the cerebrospinal fluid (CSF) may support the diagnosis of encephalitis.

Such an illness may appear one to three weeks after well-known exanthematous disorders such as rubella, varicella, infectious mononucleosis (glandular fever), Coxsacksie or ECHO virus infections.

This disorder will be characterised by a cerebellar ataxia. The patient may prefer to lie quietly in bed because sitting up with the truncal ataxia will be troublesome. Examination will detect evidence of upper limb ataxia with impaired finger-nose-finger movements, hypotonia, possibly dysarthric speech, and nystagmus. Fortunately, most patients make a complete recovery within a few weeks. In a few there will be a persisting abnormality of gait, speech, and upper limb function.

CHRONIC CEREBELLAR ATAXIA

Non-progressive ataxia

Some metabolic disorders may have their primary influence upon cerebellar function. Frequent and severe hypoglycaemia may not only cause cerebral but also cerebellar dysfunction. Hartnup disease (an impaired absorption and metabolism of tryptophan) and one of the variants of maple-syrup urine disease (which is another abnormality of amino acid metabolism) may cause intermittent cerebellar ataxia. In the former there will be a pellagra-like skin lesion, while in the latter the intermittent ataxia may be accompanied by lethargy and convulsions and be precipitated by an intercurrent infection. Lead poisoning in a child may cause generalised brain dysfunction but sometimes presents as an isolated ataxia.

Various malformations of the cerebellum give rise to non-progressive ataxia. Many of these children are unhelpfully labelled as having ataxic cerebral palsy. A reference to this has been made in Chapter 7.

The Dandy-Walker malformation is due to a blockage of the

outflow of CSF from the fourth ventricle of the brain, causing dilatation of that ventricle and hydrocephalus. While the symptoms and signs of this condition are predominantly those of hydrocephalus, ataxia is also present. The ataxia is caused by pressure on the cerebellum. Surgical treatment is a practical consideration.

Marinesco-Sjögren disease

This is characterised by spinocerebellar ataxia, as well as nystagmus, cataracts, and severe mental retardation. It is rare and appears to be autosomally recessively inherited. Therefore, there is a one in four chance of further affected infants being born to parents who already have an affected child.

Progressive ataxia

FRIEDREICH'S ATAXIA

This was first described in 1863 by the physician whose name is now linked with the condition. The principal characteristics are those of ataxia, nystagmus, kypho-scoliosis, and pes cavus. Together with this there is involvement of heart muscle producing a myocarditis or cardiomyopathy. The onset may well be within the first decade or perhaps later. Earlier presentation is more common when the condition is recessively inherited, whereas if the genetic pattern is that of a dominant inheritance (which is rare) then the onset tends to be at a later age.

Ataxia of gait is usually the earliest presentation and may be noticeable from soon after the onset of walking. The ataxia is not entirely due to cerebellar dysfunction but also to the degeneration of the posterior columns of the spinal cord that are responsible for transmitting vibration and position sense. The cerebellar ataxia and co-ordination difficulty is further aggravated by this loss of position sense. The patient will be able to stand with his eyes open, but when they are closed there will be a tendency to fall—a positive Romberg's sign. With progression of the disease there is further clinical evidence of involvement of the long motor descending tracts of the spinal cord, the pyramidal fibres, producing added weakness and spasticity.

Although there is some variability, progression is characteristic of this disorder. Peripheral nerve involvement will produce an increasing weakness. Deteriorating cerebellar dysfunction will interfere with not only gait but also arm function, speech, and swallowing. Retinitis pigmentosa and optic atrophy may occur.

Apart from the strong association with diabetes mellitus other biochemical abnormalities have been identified. Life span is limited by the cardiac abnormality, which most often results in death in young adulthood.

ROUSSY-LÉVY SYNDROME

This may or may not be a clinical entity in which several features of Friedreich's ataxia co-exist with those of Charcot-Marie-Tooth disease (Chapter 14).

ATAXIA-TELANGIECTASIA

In the young child this is often difficult to distinguish from Friedreich's ataxia. The principal features are those of a progressive ataxia of early onset, marked chorea, an undue susceptibility to infections because of immunological impairment, and the later development of cutaneous abnormalities—telangiectasia on the conjunctiva, ears, and skin flexures (Fig. 15/1). Early diagnosis is difficult because the telangiectasia often appears after a long delay. Examination of patients with ataxia-telangiectasia commonly reveals characteristic difficulty in eye movement (an oculomotor apraxia), but there is no evidence of a proprioceptive disorder as in Friedreich's ataxia.

Investigations include a search for any evidence of immunological impairment, and the detection of raised level of alphafetoprotein in the blood. A strong association exists between ataxia telangiectasia and various malignant disorders.

The neurological deterioration is variable but death inevitably

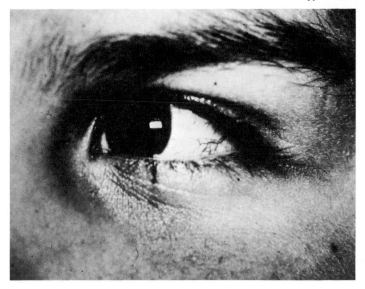

Fig. 15/1 Ataxia telangiectasia

follows probably from an infection or malignant disease. Inheritance is autosomally recessive and at present there is no totally reliable means of antenatal diagnosis.

METACHROMATIC LEUKODYSTROPHY

This condition has been discussed in detail in Chapter 8. Metachromatic leukodystrophy is a degenerative disorder due to the abnormal storage of sulphatides in the central and peripheral nervous system. There are various clinical presentations of this disorder which includes that of a progressive ataxia early in the second year of life. Progression is with a rapid increase in the ataxia, together with weakness and dementia. There is no available treatment.

Very rare causes of progressive ataxia will include abetalipoproteinaemia, in which gastro-intestinal symptoms co-exist with the findings of abnormal lipoproteins and red blood cells. In Refsum's disease ataxia is associated with a neuropathy, eczema, retinitis pigmentosa, and deafness due to an abnormality of phytanic-acid metabolism. This condition may be amenable to treatment with a low phytanic-acid diet.

In any child with progressive ataxia the possibility of a tumour must be seriously considered. Most brain tumours in children are in the posterior fossa and will present not only as signs of raised intracranial pressure but also as ataxia. The nature of this ataxia will vary and depend on the extent, site, and type of the tumour. The cerebellar astrocytomas are often situated in one hemisphere and, therefore, the signs will be unilateral; whereas the ependymomas and medulloblastomas, which are midline in origin, will have signs which suggest a midline lesion.

This chapter has discussed only some of the causes of ataxia in childhood. It is incomplete, but at least it shows that the symptom of ataxia demands very careful consideration and evaluation, as the diagnostic possibilities are moderately wide.

FURTHER READING

Gordon, N. (1976). *Paediatric Neurology for the Clinician*. Spastics International Medical Publications. Clinics in Developmental Medicine No 59/60. William Heinemann Medical Books Ltd, London.

Jabbour, J. T. et al (1973). *Paediatric Neurology Handbook*. Henry Kimpton Publishers, London.

Menkes, J. H. (1974). *Textbook of Child Neurology*, 2nd edition. Lea and Febiger Co, Philadelphia.

Till, K. (1975). *Paediatric Neurosurgery for Paediatricians and Neurosurgeons*. Blackwell Scientific Publications Limited, Oxford.

16. Mental retardation

Mental retardation may be defined as impaired intellectual functioning compared with the normal. The severity of this will vary. The accepted classification is broadly into two major groups—*severe mental retardation*, in which the intelligence quotient (IQ) will be below 50, and *moderate (or mild) mental retardation*, in which the IQ will be between 50 and 70.

Mental retardation is common. Severe mental retardation has an incidence of about four per 1 000 live births. Moderate mental retardation is about three times more common, i.e. 12 per 1 000 live births.

The first task in assessing a child recognised as being mentally retarded should be an attempt to define a specific diagnosis. Such a diagnosis may afford the opportunity to offer treatment, prognosis, and genetic advice. Careful examination may reveal a number of findings that, taken together, might suggest a specific diagnosis. Such a diagnosis may be referred to as a 'syndrome diagnosis' because it depends on the identification of a group of symptoms or signs.

In about half of the patients with severe mental retardation there may be an identifiable 'medical' diagnosis to explain the retardation. This is far less common in those with moderate mental retardation.

Many neurological disorders in childhood are associated with mental retardation of varying severity and in this book many references have been made to such associations. This chapter is concerned with several disorders that are strongly connected with mental retardation. However, it has to be recognised that in 50 per cent of children with severe mental retardation and many more who have less severe mental retardation there is no identifiable cause. Nevertheless, specific relationships are recognised in many situations.

The transmission of infection by the mother to the fetus is well recognised as a cause of syndromes associated with mental retardation. Examples of these are rubella, syphilis, cytomegalovirus and toxoplasmosis. Similarly, the ingestion of drugs may pose a risk to the normal development of the fetus, for example, the anticonvulsant phenytoin (Epanutin), and the anticancer drug methotrexate. Maternal alcoholism is associated with the so-called *fetal alcohol syndrome*, of which mental retardation is but one of the features.

Abnormalities of pregnancy such as bleeding, toxaemia, poor fetal growth, complications of delivery, and prematurity may be the cause of mental retardation.

Even after birth the very young infant is at risk from many factors that can impair brain development such as infections (particularly meningitis), hypothermia, low blood sugar and respiratory problems. In some cases metabolic disorders have an adverse effect upon brain development.

In Chapter 5 chromosomal disorders were discussed in detail. These disorders, which include Down's syndrome, are recognised as contributing significantly to specific causes of mental retardation. Down's syndrome alone is responsible for 30 per cent of known causes of severe mental retardation.

The disorders to be discussed in this chapter are a group known as the neurocutaneous syndromes and some examples of other rare syndromes strongly associated with mental retardation.

NEUROCUTANEOUS SYNDROMES (PHAKOMATOSES)

Several disorders are commonly recognised as coming under this general heading and include tuberous sclerosis, neurofibromatosis, the Sturge-Weber syndrome, von Hippel-Lindau syndrome, and ataxia telangiectasia. The unifying feature is that they all have some disorder of the nervous system and the skin.

Tuberous sclerosis (epiloia, adenoma sebaceum, or Bourneville's disease)

Clinically, tuberous sclerosis (TS) is associated with three principal features—epilepsy, mental retardation, and skin lesions known as adenoma sebaceum (Fig. 16/1).

Patients with this condition may have numerous very small tumours or lumps growing in all their body tissues—the skin, brain, heart, kidneys, liver and lungs.

It is the small tumours, or fibromata, that commonly are seen on the cheeks that constitute the so-called *adenoma sebaceum.* These adenomata are not seen in the very young child but develop

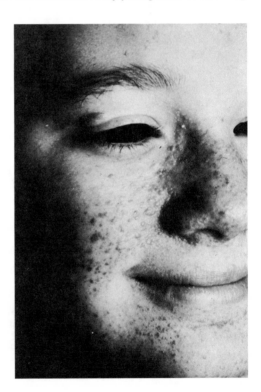

Fig. 16/1
Tuberous sclerosis

in the first few years of life. They form the most well-known skin features of this condition but are not the only cutaneous signs. Pale, depigmented patches of the skin may be found. In the infant a very careful look for such patches may have to be undertaken with the aid of ultraviolet light using a Wood's filter. Thickened areas of skin reminiscent of orange peel—shagreen patches—can commonly be seen in the lumbar sacral region. Areas of brown staining—café-au-lait patches, little fibromata under the skin and toe nails 'subungual fibromata' are found in patients with TS. The two principal features of epilepsy and mental retardation are due to small tumour-like masses (glial tumours) in the brain. These glial tumours contain calcium which may show up on plain skull x-rays or on a brain scan. There is a common association of TS with severe epilepsy in early infancy—the infantile spasms syndrome.

Classically, this condition is associated with the triad of epilepsy, mental retardation, and adenoma sebaceum but it is recognised that not all the three problems may exist in every affected patient. Forty per cent ultimately have the skin features; only 60 per cent are mentally retarded, although most have epilepsy. There is an immense variation between the severity of epilepsy and the degree of mental retardation in affected individuals.

The outlook is variable. In many there is general progressive mental deterioration with age, possibly because of the sometimes very severe epilepsy. The presence of tumours in the heart, kidney, or brain increase the mortality, especially when they are of significant size or malignant change occurs.

The condition is dominantly inherited but often from parents who may have minimal features of the condition. Tuberous sclerosis, however, is recognised as having a high mutation rate so that the individuals affected, while able to transmit it to their offspring, may not have inherited it from their own parents. Clearly, when the diagnosis is made parents should be examined for the stigmata of the disorder so that risks to future offspring may be recognised.

Von Recklinghausen's disease (neurofibromatosis)

Small cutaneous tumours and numerous flat café-au-lait skin patches are the diagnostic features of this condition. Again, various tumours may occur in other tissues or organs, e.g. the central or peripheral nervous system, bones, muscles, and endocrine glands.

The tumours that may be seen in the skin are neurofibromata and are obviously related to nerves. As well as the tumours in the cutaneous nerves, there appears to be a tendency towards similar growth in the optic nerve, the auditory nerve, and the meningeal coverings of the brain and spinal cord. In some patients the principal clinical findings will be the café-au-lait patches that appear early in infancy while in others the two features, patches and cutaneous tumours, co-exist. Other abnormalities associated with von Recklinghausen's disease include hypertrophy of extremities or parts of the body, malignant changes, various bone abnormalities, endocrine abnormalities, and also tumours of the medulla of the adrenal glands—phaeochromocytoma. About half the patients with von Recklinghausen's disease may develop some neurological symptoms and five to ten per cent may develop malignant disease.

Mental retardation is three times as common as in the population as a whole, although the reason for this is not fully understood. Seizures often occur and may be associated with a brain tumour.

There is no specific treatment, although when any of the tumours do produce difficulties then treatment will be that most appropriate to the type and site of the tumour.

Sturge-Weber syndrome

A port-wine stain (a cutaneous haemangioma) of one side of the face, commonly associated with a hemiplegia on the other side, mental subnormality, and epilepsy are the hallmarks of the Sturge-Weber syndrome (Fig. 16/2). In some cases the skin

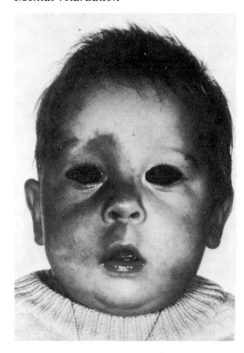

Fig. 16/2
Sturge Weber syndrome

lesion may be more extensive. Buphthalmos (bull's eye), which is an intense increase in pressure of the eye at birth due to the lack of drainage of fluid from inside the eye, is also found.

In the brain, on the same side as the facial skin lesion, there will be an abnormal development of the blood vessels on the surface of the brain, particularly in the occipital and parietal areas—leptomeningeal angiomatosis. Calcium will be deposited in these abnormal vessels and sometimes show up on the x-rays of the skull with a characteristic 'railroad track' appearance of double contour lines.

Ninety per cent of patients with Sturge-Weber syndrome have epilepsy, 30 per cent are mentally retarded and 30 to 40 per cent have a hemiplegia on the side opposite to the haemangioma.

Control of the epilepsy may be difficult and at times hemispherectomy (removal of a cerebral hemisphere) has to be undertaken.

This condition is not genetically determined.

Specific syndrome diagnosis (based on dysmorphic features)

In these syndromes—some examples of which are given below—the diagnosis will be suggested purely on the basis of a collection of clinical findings. The genetic pattern of inheritance may be well known, although no chromosomal or metabolic disorder is known to be associated.

In any single case of such a syndrome it is unusual in an individual patient to have all the features ascribed to the syndrome. Diagnosis can reasonably be made if most of the common features are present. Inevitably, total diagnostic certainty cannot always exist.

LAURENCE-MOON-BIEDL SYNDROME

The principal features of this rare recessively inherited condition are mental retardation, retinitis pigmentosa (a degeneration of the retina producing initially night blindness and then total visual loss), obesity, small genitalia, and polydactyly (extra fingers or toes). There is a further strong association with deafness and with heart disease. The condition is easy to diagnose if all the five cardinal features are present, but it is believed that the syndrome may exist when only one or two such features are present and also that it can exist with other features such as optic atrophy rather than the retinitis pigmentosa.

It is important to be sure of the diagnosis of Laurence-Moon-Biedl syndrome so that parents may be given genetic advice.

CORNELIA-DE-LANGE'S SYNDROME (AMSTERDAM DWARF)

Although rare, this may be more common than previously suspected. Mental retardation is invariable and most commonly severe, although cases do occur when the retardation is relatively mild and the specific diagnostic features are less marked.

Most patients with Cornelia-de-Lange's syndrome are small at birth and remain small, often have a growl-like cry, and are particularly hairy with eyebrows meeting in the middle (synophrys). The space between the bottom of the nose and the upper lip is large and the lips themselves are thin and have a downward curve at the angle of the mouth. The thumbs are unusually sited, being apparently nearer the wrist than usual and various other abnormalities of the shape and size of the hands and the skin creases are often seen. The feet are often very small (micromelia) and some of the toes may be joined together (syndactyly). Not only are most of the children with the Cornelia-de-Lange's syndrome severely retarded, but self-destructive mutilating behaviour is common. This syndrome is apparently not genetically determined, although reports do exist of its recurrence within a family and the finding of chromosomal abnormalities in some patients.

INCONTINENTIA PIGMENTI SYNDROME (BLOCH-SULZBERGER DISEASE)

This disorder may be X linked and in the affected males lethal at birth so that only heterozygote females survive. The diagnosis of incontinentia pigmenti syndrome is based upon characteristic skin lesions, which may be present from infancy. From an initial inflammatory or vesicular type of skin lesion the progression is towards pigmentation over large areas of the body. A third of such patients are mentally retarded and an equal proportion have delayed mental development. Alopecia, various eye abnormalities, and skeletal abnormalities are common. As the condition may be sex linked it has been suggested that mothers of affected children should be carefully examined for any minor skin manifestations of the disorder.

APERT'S SYNDROME (ACROCEPHALOSYNDACTYLY)

The principal features of this disorder are that affected children have short but high heads, prominent eyes, and varying degrees of syndactyly of the toes and fingers. Mental retardation is common but not invariably associated with this syndrome and the severity of this may not necessarily be marked.

The genetic pattern is an autosomal dominant, although the majority occur as fresh mutations. An association between this condition and a high paternal age has been suggested.

RUBINSTEIN-TAYBI SYNDROME

This is often difficult to diagnose as the salient features may be somewhat difficult to identify. Mental retardation is very common, together with several facial features that include downward-slanting eyes, a beaked nose with the septum extending down below the nostrils, and low-slung and malformed ears. The most consistent findings, however, are broad, unusually angulated thumbs. Small or absent genitalia (cryptorchidism) are very common. As with Cornelia-de-Lange's syndrome, partially because of the difficulty in making a diagnosis, it is possibly more common than has previously been suspected.

The Rubinstein-Taybi syndrome does not appear to be a genetically determined disorder.

SMITH-LEMLI-OPITZ SYNDROME

This rare autosomal recessive disorder is invariably associated with mental retardation and often with poor growth, floppiness, microcephaly with a narrow frontal area, droopy eyelids (ptosis), and slanted or low-set ears. A single palmar (simian) skin crease is common and cryptorchidism and other genital abnormalities are often seen in the male. Several other associations have also been reported and include seizures, heart defects, cataracts, and syndactyly of the second and third toes. The diagnosis is more commonly made in males, probably because of the genital abnormalities rendering the diagnosis easier to make.

RILEY-DAY SYNDROME (FAMILIAL DYSAUTONOMIA)

The many and various clinical features are indicative of autonomic nervous system dysfunction. Half of the affected individuals are mentally retarded and half have epilepsy. Infants do not thrive. Swallowing difficulties, aspiration pneumonias and cyclical vomiting occur commonly. The most well-known clinical features of Riley-Day syndrome are due to the autonomic dysfunction: abnormal sweating, skin blotching, insensitivity to pain, lack of tear formation (severe enough to cause corneal scarring), taste deficiency, unstable temperature, labile blood pressure, urinary frequency, and absent tendon reflexes. The aspiration pneumonia and cardiac disorders pose a serious threat to survival and many children die before the age of 10 years.

The genetic pattern is that of an autosomal recessive condition and the condition is more common in Ashkanazim Jews.

SOTOS SYNDROME (CEREBRAL GIGANTISM)

It is not known why children with Sotos syndrome do have such marked growth and doubt exists as to whether all of those diagnosed as having this syndrome do really have a single specific aetiology. Over 80 per cent of these children are mentally retarded. They are large at birth and also have large heads and feet. There is a prominent forehead (dolichocephaly), downward-slanting eyes, hyperteleorism, a large chin, a high palate, and coarse facial features. Growth rate in the early years is excessive but a slowing down later may result in the ultimate adult height being near normal. This is not a genetically determined disease.

MINOR MALFORMATIONS OR ANOMALIES

Minor malformations or anomalies are common in all individuals and estimates have suggested that 14 per cent of newborn babies have at least one minor anomaly. However, the greater the number of such anomalies the greater will be the chance of a co-existing major malformation. If three minor anomalies are detected there will be a 90 per cent chance of a major anomaly also being present. Therefore, in routine clinical examination a search for all such anomalies is important.

These will include abnormalities of skin creases (particularly a single palmar crease), the shapes of the fingers and the toes, unusually large fontanelles, inner epicanthic folds, hyperteleorism, downward-slanting eyes, abnormal shape and position of the ears, unusual hair patterning, and abnormalities of the genitalia. With many of these abnormalities their presence is a familial phenomenon and it is important to exclude the presence of any of these in either parent.

The number of syndromes in which mental retardation is an important feature is very large indeed but in only a few children with mental retardation can a specific syndrome be clinically diagnosed. Nevertheless, a careful, comprehensive physical examination is vital in all.

Because of the very large number of syndromes relevant to mental retardation, which are often individually quite rare, a number of reference texts and atlases exist. These will contain photographs and summaries of the clinical features of many of the disorders. These are extremely useful as an aid to clinical practice.

FURTHER READING

Emery, A. E. H. (1979). *Elements of Medical Genetics*, 5th edition. Churchill Livingstone, Edinburgh.

Kirman, B. and Bicknell, J. (1975). *Mental Handicap*. Churchill Livingstone, Edinburgh.

MacKay, R. I. (1976). *Mental Handicap in Child Health Practice*. Volume in the Postgraduate Paediatric Series (General editor, Apley, J.). Butterworths, London.

Smith, D. W. (1976). *Recognisable Patterns of Human Malformation*, 2nd edition. Volume VII in series Major Problems in Clinical Pediatrics (Ed Schaffer, A.). W. B. Saunders Co, Philadelphia.

17. Epilepsy

Epilepsy is one of the commonest neurological disorders in child-hood, but despite this it is often misunderstood, misdiagnosed, and mismanaged.

The incidence is difficult to estimate but a suggestion has been made that about eight in every 1 000 children under the age of five years will have one or more seizures.

An epileptic attack is due to a transitory disturbance of the function of the brain. Epilepsy is accepted as a paroxysmal and transitory disturbance of the brain owing to an *excessive neuronal discharge* which is likely to develop suddenly, cease spontane-ously, and show a tendency to recur. Epilepsy is not a specific disease.

There are many differing forms of epilepsy, and the clinical dissimilarity between them is quite striking; classification is difficult. A simple division is to consider epilepsy to be either *partial* or *generalised*.

The *partial epilepsies* include Jacksonian focal epilepsies in which a seizure may involve only one part of the body—very commonly one side; and some of the psychomotor or temporal lobe seizures, when certain behavioural changes take place as a major manifestation of the attack. The *generalised epilepsies* include forms of absence attacks including petit mal epilepsy, tonic-clonic attacks (grand mal), akinetic 'drop attacks', generalised myoclonic attacks, and infantile spasms.

DIAGNOSIS

There are several conditions which can easily be confused with epilepsy in childhood. These include hypoglycaemia, habitual

spasm or tic, breath-holding attacks, migraine, benign paroxysmal vertigo, syncope, tetany, and hysterical or simulated
attacks. Such conditions must be identified when investigating a
child with recurrent episodes of an unknown nature, as the diagnosis of epilepsy carries major implications for the child, the
parents, and teachers.

Diagnosis depends almost entirely upon a careful history
obtained from as many witnesses as possible and, in part, the
patient. It is necessary to know the frequency, duration, charac-
ter, timing, and possible precipitating factors of any attack. Any
abnormality of eye movement during an attack is important to
note. Enquiries should be made as to whether there is any aura or
warning of an impending attack and incontinence, tongue biting,
injury, or changes in complexion during an attack. The state of
the patient immediately after an attack should be known.

Any patient presenting with possible epilepsy needs to undergo
a thorough examination by a doctor.

The role of special investigations to confirm the clinical diagnosis of epilepsy in childhood is controversial. Investigations may
be important in defining which form of epilepsy may be present,
and also in looking for a possible cause, although in many this will
never be known and the term idiopathic is used.

Radiology

The skull x-ray will be normal in most children. Occasionally,
calcified areas, due either to previous cerebral infections, early
tuberous sclerosis (see Chapter 16), or a slow-growing tumour,
may be seen. There may be an inequality in the size of the middle
cranial fossae, consequent upon long-standing atrophy of one
temporal lobe; this would support the diagnosis of temporal lobe
epilepsy. Raised intracranial pressure (Chapter 12) will be apparent from the appearance of a plain skull x-ray. More detailed
neuroradiological studies may be carried out if there is a clinical
indication, using either a CAT scan or angiographic studies (see
Chapter 3).

Electroencephalography (EEG)

This is an amplification and recording of the electrical activity of the brain over about 20 to 30 minutes, with a series of electrodes attached to the scalp and head. Over the years much has been learnt about the basic rhythms and characteristics of these electrical waves in health and disease. However, the 'usefulness' of EEG recordings in the diagnosis of epilepsy can be guaranteed to provoke a brisk debate among groups of paediatricians and groups of neurologists! Patients with definite seizures may have a normal EEG (see Fig. 3/13, p. 54) while patients who have never had a seizure may have an 'epileptic' EEG (see Fig. 3/14, p. 54). Whatever view is taken, there is a general agreement of the need to correlate EEG findings as much as possible with the clinical features of any patient. (I believe that an EEG can be helpful in occasionally diagnosing an epileptic disorder, characterising the type of seizure, and managing some types of status epilepticus.)

Electroencephalographic telemetry, in which recordings are made in a mobile patient over a period of time, and various techniques by which EEG signals are stored and analysed by using an on-line computer, are new developments that are beginning to find clinical usefulness.

Biochemical investigations

These may be important in a few patients whose seizures are due to primary biochemical disorders. It is particularly relevant in the neonate because of the risk of hypoglycaemia and hypocalcaemia. Fasting estimations of blood sugar, calcium, and magnesium frequently need to be considered in the younger child. In a small number of patients, particularly those with infantile onset of seizures, more unusual biochemical abnormalities may exist which are inborn errors of metabolism. If such disorders are suspected biochemical investigations may need to be extensive. Although unlikely, the possibility of lead poisoning must always be borne in mind.

Other investigations

Congenital or acquired infections of the central nervous system
are sometimes responsible for seizure disorders and, when this is
thought appropriate, bacterial, viral, and serological investigations are considered.

SEIZURES IN THE NEONATAL PERIOD

Seizures are common in the neonatal period but because of their
often uncharacteristic presentation they may be difficult to recognise. They can manifest as 'twitching', 'jitteriness', apnoea, or
irregular respirations. All persons who care for neonates must be
constantly on the alert for any of these signs.

Birth trauma

Cerebral haemorrhage or severe asphyxia may produce seizures
soon after birth. The occurrence of seizures in such an infant has
been shown to generally carry a poor prognosis.

Biochemical upsets

Hypoglycaemia, especially in a premature or 'small-for-dates'
infant, is common and must be recognised quickly and treated
appropriately to avoid long-term damage. Hypocalcaemia, and
occasionally hypomagnesaemia, may occur typically at five days
of life in bottle-fed babies and cause seizures which are easily
treated. Reference has already been made to biochemical disorders due to inborn errors of metabolism.

Pyridoxine (vitamin B$_6$) dependency

This is an exceedingly rare but easily treated cause of neonatal
seizures (Chapter 9). The regular giving of pyridoxine during

infancy is curative. With this condition the mother may often believe that seizures were occurring even in the uterus.

SEIZURES IN LATER INFANCY

Infantile spasms (West syndrome, 'salaam' attacks)

This is a very serious form of myoclonic epilepsy of infancy. In some patients in which spasms develop, there may be a known pre-existing neurological abnormality; but in others, neurological development up to that time was thought normal. The latter group is often referred to as *cryptogenic*. With the onset of spasms there is commonly a marked regression and loss of previously attained developmental milestones.

Infantile spasms cause the infant to 'bend' suddenly and to have repeated frequent 'showers' of flexions. Occasionally these 'showers' may be extensions of the whole body as opposed to flexions. The flexion episodes are often called 'salaam' attacks and are more common on waking. A mistaken diagnosis of colic is all too often made when the spasms first occur.

The EEG is always abnormal and an abnormality commonly seen is known as hypsarrhythmia.

A few conditions have been linked with the infantile spasm syndrome. These include some metabolic disorders, tuberous sclerosis (epiloia), and some infections of the central nervous system. In the search for a cause, despite these associations, extensive investigations most often give negative results.

The outlook for normal mental development and long-term freedom from seizures is generally poor.

Febrile seizures

These are associated with a rapid rise in body temperature, most commonly due to viral infections. They are most prevalent between the ages of six months and five years. Most seizures are short but tend to recur. A family history of febrile seizures is common. The cause of the fever must be considered to ensure that it is not a consequence of the seizure itself. Prolonged febrile seizures may be associated with the development of temporal lobe epilepsy in later life.

SEIZURES IN LATER CHILDHOOD

Tonic-clonic attacks (grand mal)

A good eye-witness account of a tonic-clonic seizure should leave little diagnostic doubt. Tonic-clonic seizures consist of a loss of consciousness and posture, stiffening (tonic phase), generalised jerking movements (clonic phase), sometimes with a cry, facial flushing, incontinence, tongue biting, and salivation from the mouth; if the seizure is in any way prolonged, there will be some cyanosis. After an attack, many patients will have a headache or backache and be sleepy. Amnesia for the event is common.

Careful clinical examination by a doctor is mandatory and may be supplemented by plain skull x-rays and later an EEG. The possibility of idiopathic hypoglycaemia is always borne in mind when a differential diagnosis is considered and a fasting blood sugar estimation is often measured. In a high proportion of patients with tonic-clonic seizures no cause will be found despite extensive investigations and careful review of all known facts. Brain tumours in children seldom present with seizures.

Petit mal seizures

This term is all too often used rather too loosely to describe all forms of 'absence' attacks. Petit mal attacks usually start between three years of age and the teens. They consist of momentary cessation of activity and awareness, and are normally associated with a characteristic EEG abnormality—3 Hertz (cycles per second) spike and wave formation. Although the individual attacks last only a few seconds, they may be frequent and interfere with school work. Some flickering of the eyes is sometimes seen but there is never any falling. Petit mal seizures are more common in girls, and carry a generally favourable prognosis.

Psychomotor or temporal lobe attacks

This form of epilepsy may sometimes be difficult to distinguish from petit mal attacks. Common presentations are as altered sensations and awareness. These altered sensations or aura can either be an abnormal taste in the mouth, a feeling of 'having been here before' (déjà vu), a smell, a peculiar abdominal sensation, fear or vertigo followed by alteration of awareness, perhaps together with some automatic behaviour. Associated behavioural problems are common and at times it is difficult to decide which is a behavioural problem and which is epileptic. From the aura, some patients rapidly go into a tonic-clonic seizure. Sometimes temporal lobe attacks may present as rage episodes, and very rarely as nightmares.

A clinical examination between attacks is usually normal, but abnormalities in the visual field are occasionally seen when there is an underlying structural lesion of the temporal lobe interfering with the optic radiations.

Skull x-rays may demonstrate an asymmetry of the middle cranial fossae due to atrophy of a temporal lobe. An EEG may be helpful in distinguishing between petit mal and temporal lobe epilepsy, especially if the patient is drowsy or asleep. The description of the attacks alone often makes differentiation of one form from the other very difficult. While a *focus* may be found on the EEG in typical psychomotor epilepsy, it could be found elsewhere than in the temporal lobes. For this reason, many doctors prefer to reserve the term temporal lobe epilepsy to those in which the temporal lobe can be definitely implicated.

Reference has already been made to the association of prolonged febrile seizures and the later development of temporal lobe epilepsy due to scarring of the medial side of the temporal lobe. Hamartomata (congenital structural tumours) or slow-growing, benign tumours in the anterior temporal lobes may be a cause of temporal lobe attacks and can sometimes be surgically removed. Temporal lobe epilepsy may sometimes be inherited.

Focal epilepsy

This may be either sensory or motor with the seizures confined to one part of the body, and often with consciousness retained. The term Jacksonian epilepsy may be used. Focal attacks may progress and spread, and end in a full tonic-clonic seizure. A focal weakness and paralysis for a variable length of time may develop after such a seizure and this is known as a Todd's paralysis.

In adults, focal epilepsy essentially implies a localised anatomical epileptogenic lesion such as a scar or tumour. Although this form of seizure is quite common in hemiplegic children a focal lesion is less commonly found in young children than it is in adults.

Myoclonic epilepsy

One variety of myoclonic epilepsy—infantile spasms syndrome—has already been described. The term *myoclonus* simply refers to involuntary, irregular jerks of muscle groups, which may be due to disorders in any number of parts of the nervous system. Thus, myoclonic jerks may be seen with tonic-clonic seizures due to a definite brain disorder or rarely as an isolated phenomenon due to a spinal cord problem. The combination of tonic-clonic seizures, drop attacks, absences, myoclonus, and often mental retardation, may be referred to as the Lennox-Gastaut syndrome or petit mal variant. In some the picture may be dominated by absences and be difficult to distinguish from other types of absence attacks. Myoclonic epilepsy in childhood presents as varying combinations of seizure types and severity. Diagnostic evaluation and prognostications are difficult.

Myoclonic epilepsy may also be seen in several neurodegenerative disorders, such as the various forms of Batten's disease, and the slow virus infection known as sub-acute sclerosing panencephalitis (see Chapter 7). A progressive familial myoclonic epilepsy occurs in which amyloid bodies (Lafora's bodies) are found on biopsy of the brain. This familial progressive myoclonic epilepsy is also sometimes known as Unverricht's myoclonic epilepsy and, as well as being associated with other seizure disorders, is usually also accompanied by a progressive dementia.

The *dancing-eyes syndrome* or *myoclonic encephalopathy of infancy* is an almost continuous myoclonic jerking of the limbs and eyes, with no evidence of seizure activity on an EEG. Despite the absence of definite seizures, these patients are often thought to have myoclonic epilepsy. There is an established association between the dancing-eyes syndrome and either occult or known neuroblastomas or ganglioneuromas.

Akinetic attacks (drop attacks)

'Drop attacks' is a very descriptive term. When they occur patients lose all tone and drop straight to the ground but recover instantly and continue as if nothing had happened. Falling to the ground without warning gives a high risk of facial and head injury. These seizures, which are a form of myoclonic epilepsy, may occur alone or in combination with other seizure types.

Epilepsia partialis continua

This is a continuous focal epilepsy, often without loss of consciousness but with appropriate focal weakness. A localised cerebral disorder may be causative and should be diligently sought. Response to medical treatment is often poor.

Reflex epilepsy

There are a large number of reflex epilepsies, the most common being the so-called *photosensitive epilepsy* or *television epilepsy*. Seizures may be induced by being close to the television in some, when the receiver is not correctly adjusted. Discotheques can pose similar problems. The photic stimulation given during the routine EEG may identify spike discharges at certain flicker rates. In some patients there may be an uncontrollable 'pull' towards the flickering television screen. Seizures or EEG spikes may be induced by just waving the fingers in front of the eyes while looking towards a bright light. Treatment with most anticonvulsants is ineffective.

PROLONGED FITS

Status epilepticus

This is a series of tonic-clonic seizures without intervening recovery of consciousness, and is a medical emergency. Continuous seizure activity will cause impairment of oxygen supply to the brain (hypoxia), brain swelling, hyperpyrexia, and death. Frequent, prolonged seizures will cause brain scarring. While a specific aetiology may not be apparent, sudden withdrawal of anticonvulsant medication can be a cause of status epilepticus. An encephalitis may start with status epilepticus.

MINOR MOTOR STATUS EPILEPTICUS

With this form of status epilepticus there is continuous minor motor seizure activity and the clinical picture may include marked mental dulling and drooling, with perhaps small jerks or twitches of the limbs or face. Minor motor status epilepticus sometimes heralds the onset of a progressive cerebral disease. Prompt medical treatment will fortunately often return a child to near normality. The EEG is a helpful investigation, as it will confirm seizure activity.

DRUG TREATMENT OF SEIZURES

The aims of therapy are to prevent seizures, or at least reduce their severity and frequency, while at the same time not interfering with the child's development. All anticonvulsants are powerful drugs, and toxic symptoms can occur. Even very small doses of anticonvulsants can be toxic in some children. The recent facility to measure blood levels of drugs has proved to be helpful in patients whose seizures have been difficult to treat and who are taking combinations of drugs. Studies of blood levels have also emphasised that treatment should begin with a single drug.

In the neonatal period, seizures due to hypocalcaemia and hypoglycaemia are treated with calcium and sugar respectively, while for other seizures in the neonate phenobarbitone (Luminal) remains the drug of choice.

The treatment of febrile seizures is somewhat problematic. The acute attack is treated by lowering the body temperature and simple first aid procedures. The prevention of recurrent attacks has been attempted with various anticonvulsants given regularly. Because of the risk of brain scarring, the question of prophylaxis is important. At present the suggested drug of choice is phenobarbitone, despite the fact that the drug may cause behavioural problems in many patients. Rectal diazepam (Valium) or intramuscular paraldehyde (possibly given by some parents after careful instruction) at the onset of an attack, however, may turn out to be the most reasonable method of ensuring that attacks are not prolonged.

Infantile spasms respond poorly to most anticonvulsants. A short course of daily high dose ACTH or steroids is often efficacious, although recently benzodiazepine drugs such as nitrazepam (Mogadon) have been found to be useful. Unfortunately, ACTH and steroids have not convincingly been shown to improve the long-term outlook after the onset of infantile spasms.

Tonic-clonic, focal motor and psychomotor attacks may respond to treatment with phenytoin (Epanutin), carbamazepine (Tegretol), or sodium valproate (Epilim).

Petit mal epilepsy is usually controlled adequately with ethosuximide (Zarontin), or sodium valproate (Epilim).

The myoclonic epilepsies in their various forms are often

difficult to treat, although the benzodiazepines (Mogadon) and sodium valproate (Epilim) may be very helpful.

A high fat and low carbohydrate diet which will render a patient ketotic (a ketogenic diet) may be used in several forms of epilepsy when there is poor response to anticonvulsant therapy or an unacceptable incidence of side-effects from medication. Despite recent modifications to this diet with the incorporation of solutions of medium-chain triglycerides, it remains for many rather unpalatable. Nevertheless, there are situations when the institution of this diet needs to be seriously considered.

Surgical treatment may be appropriate in a very small number of patients who have evidence to support a structural lesion in the anterior temporal lobe. Selection for such procedures is difficult and should be considered only after all attempts at medical treatment have failed.

Status epilepticus and minor motor status epilepticus often respond to a slow intravenous injection of diazepam (Valium). If needed, this can also be given as an infusion. Chlormethiazole (Heminevrin 0.8%) infusion may also be helpful, as may a short course of steroids. Patients with status epilepticus that is difficult to treat need careful observation, preferably in an intensive care ward. Fluid and electrolyte balance, temperature control, and respiratory function all need careful monitoring.

There is more to the treatment of epilepsy in children than the prescription of anticonvulsants. This alone may be complicated because of the growth and maturation of children so that a static situation seldom exists. Medication requirements inevitably vary as a child grows and is exposed to a varying environment.

Many parents are terrified when they first see their child in a seizure and feel that the child is about to die. In addition, society has an aversion and fear of epilepsy. The fears of parents and the reservations of society need to be recognised and discussed, not only with the parents but with school teachers and others involved with child care. Most important is that parents and teachers need to know basic first-aid so that they are able to cope with the child should there be another seizure. Parents also have fears about the effects of medication on their children. Now that so much is known about the deleterious effects of certain anticonvulsants on concentration and learning, it is important to discuss parents' fears with them; in any such discussions teachers should be included.

Children with seizure disorders should not be over-protected. While some with attacks that are difficult to control need to wear protective helmets, others need only be restricted by not allowing climbing to great heights, swimming unsupervised, and cycling on the road or in a public place.

The outlook for cessation of attacks is always uncertain in an individual child, although in most children with febrile, tonic-clonic, petit mal, and uncomplicated akinetic seizures, the outlook for easily achievable control is good. A good initial response to anticonvulsants is encouraging when considering prognosis.

Continued medication for at least two years is the generally accepted rule, but avoiding sudden withdrawal of medication or withdrawal during puberty.

The risks of siblings developing epilepsy or of the patient having offspring with epilepsy is often asked. It is impossible to give a single answer to the hereditary risks that cover all the different forms of epilepsy, some of which are, in any case, secondary to other specific conditions. Counselling for epilepsy has always to be undertaken with extreme caution. All of us have some threshold at which, if stimulated appropriately, we will convulse, and in some individuals this threshold may be particularly low. It is this that might be genetically determined.

The needs of children with epilepsy are many and various. From time to time the children and their families are likely to require all the resources and patience that can be mustered from those members of the caring professions with whom they come into contact.

FURTHER READING

Laidlaw, J. and Richens, A. (Jt Eds) (1976). *A Textbook of Epilepsy*. Churchill Livingstone, Edinburgh.

O'Donohue, N. V. (1979). *Epilepsies of Childhood*. Butterworths, London.

Scott, D. (1976). *Understanding EEG. An Introduction to Electro-encephalography*. Duckworth and Co Ltd, London.

18. Migraine

Migraine is a familial disorder traditionally characterised by recurrent attacks of headache which can be widely variable in intensity, frequency, and duration. It may occur in infants and children and is more common than epilepsy. It is difficult to diagnose in the younger child because not only is the presentation often unusual but the history vague.

The cause of migraine is uncertain. Attacks consist of two phases: constriction, usually of the cerebral blood vessels, followed by dilatation. The precipitating mechanism is unknown but various physical and emotional triggers have been implicated in individual patients, such as stress, food, or drugs. A family history may often be obtained.

Classification of migraine is difficult because it presents in different ways and at any age—the only common feature being the episodic nature of the attacks. One classification is as follows:

1. Classical migraine
2. Complicated migraine
3. Migraine equivalents

CLASSICAL MIGRAINE

Classical migraine may start long before puberty, when it is more common in boys than girls; after puberty the reverse is the case.

The initial constrictive phase may be associated with various visual distortions, transient scotomata (blind spots), flashing lights, and micropsia (objects looking smaller than normal). Naturally, in the young child it would be unusual to obtain an exact history of such phenomena. More usual would be a history of episodes of misery, inactivity, and perhaps pallor. The dilatory phase of an attack will be characterised by severe bilateral or unilateral headache and vomiting, usually lasting at least half an hour. Many patients prefer to lie down in a dark room during an attack; if they manage to sleep the headache may well have eased on waking. Physical examination is normal, although scalp tenderness is occasionally found.

With a clear history of visual phenomena followed by headache, nausea, and vomiting, there should seldom be any difficulty in making a diagnosis of migraine. In some patients tension headaches may be a more appropriate diagnosis, particularly if there is identifiable stress. It must be remembered though that stress often aggravates migraine, so the distinction from tension headaches may be difficult.

Intracranial pathology must be excluded by careful clinical examination. A very rare cause of a syndrome remarkably like migraine may be a form of hyperammonaemia (Chapter 9).

COMPLICATED MIGRAINE

Hemiplegic migraine, ophthalmoplegic migraine, and basilar migraine are the better-known examples of complicated migraine. They occur as often in children as in adults. In these forms of migraine the clinical picture is due to the over-riding effects of constricted vasculature. Headache is not an invariable feature of these attacks. The diagnosis is difficult to make when only one attack has occurred. In each case a most careful clinical evaluation must be undertaken and often neurological investigations will be necessary to exclude other diagnoses, particularly brain tumours.

Hemiplegic migraine may start in infancy and involve different sides in different attacks. Recovery is normally over hours but may be over days. Aphasia (loss of speech) may occur. Very rarely, recovery from a hemiplegia may be incomplete.

Ophthalmoplegic migraine virtually always affects one or other third cranial nerve, producing ptosis (drooping of the lid) and paralysis of the constrictor muscles of the pupil and some of the extra-ocular muscles, causing a squint. As with hemiplegic migraine, recovery takes place over hours or days.

Basilar migraine may produce a complicated neurological picture due to brainstem ischaemia. Vomiting is common, with paraesthesia around the mouth, tinnitus, disorders of eye movements, ataxia, and even hallucinations due to temporal lobe ischaemia.

MIGRAINE EQUIVALENTS

Abdominal migraine, cyclical vomiting (periodic syndrome), and benign paroxysmal vertigo may be examples of so-called migraine equivalents. In many cases there will be a positive family history of migraine and the more classical features of migraine will probably emerge with increasing age.

The relationship between migraine and epilepsy is well established. The diagnostic difficulty is always in deciding whether a transient hemiplegia is a post-ictal Todd's paralysis (Chapter 17) or if it is due to hemiplegic migraine. Patients with migraine are also at greater risk than the population at large of having epileptic seizures. The reverse is also true—migraine is more common in patients who are known epileptics.

General management

Suspicious provoking factors, whether dietary, occupational, or emotional, should be identified and removed.

If lying in a darkened room is insufficient to abort or relieve an attack of classical migraine, analgesics, preferably mild ones, should be given early in the attack. Anti-emetics, either given by injection or suppository, may be required. Ergotamine is a vasoconstrictor and may be helpful with the headache of classical migraine; it is potentially dangerous when used in the vasoconstrictive phase of complicated migraine.

Several drugs have been used in the attempted prophylaxis of migraine with varying degrees of success. As yet no one agent has emerged as more helpful than the others. Propranolol, flufenamic acid, antihistamines, amitryptiline, 5-hydroxytryptamine antagonists, clonidine and carbamazepine are some of the many agents that appear to help some patients for some of the time.

Most important in the management of migraine is a careful initial assessment and equally careful re-assessment of the patient (rather than the condition alone) and the family. Removal of the anxiety of a more sinister diagnosis may in itself be highly therapeutic. The long-term outlook in migraine is very uncertain, although most patients may enjoy long periods without attacks.

FURTHER READING

Brown, J. K. (1977). Migraine and Migraine Equivalents in Children. *Developmental Medicine and Child Neurology.* **1**, 683.

19. Learning and behavioural disorders

Children with learning and behavioural disorders may often be referred to paediatric neurologists so that any underlying neurological disorder or dysfunction can be assessed.

Learning disorders are of two types: those caused by a generalised slowness to learn, and those of a more specific nature where the learning difficulty can be defined as hampering progress in an identifiable area or areas.

Behavioural disorders are identified and diagnosed when a child repeatedly and persistently behaves in a manner unacceptable to his social group. These may be restricted to certain situations such as school, home, or hospital. In diagnosing a child as having a behavioural disorder, care has to be taken in distinguishing those situations where the child's behaviour is as a direct result of a disturbed family background or an underlying learning disability.

In all the disorders discussed previously in this book the importance of a careful history and examination has been stressed. In most disorders it has been stated that the diagnosis can usually be made accurately from a history with the examination and necessary investigations providing confirmation.

In the group of disorders described in this chapter the problem of diagnosis is often very difficult; and although the contribution of different health service workers has been referred to, in this group the multidisciplinary team is essential to make an accurate diagnosis. The importance of a social history and the identification of the stress factors present need to be carefully recorded and investigated. Together with this, the child's past health and any disability or handicaps must be carefully assessed in relation to all spheres of the child's situation—social, intellectual, emotional, and practical.

The most common learning and behavioural disorders are discussed in a superficial way in this chapter; it is not intended to provide a comprehensive picture of learning and behavioural disorders, but rather to stress the importance of a link between some disorders and neurological disease.

Chapters 6 and 16 have specifically discussed mental retardation, although many other conditions described have been noted to be strongly associated with retardation. Children who are mentally retarded may occasionally, because of delay in the recognition of their severe mental retardation, present for the first time when they start school. Very often these children will, because of the inability to cope with the acquisition of the necessary skills, be thought to have a specific learning or behavioural disorder. No further consideration will be given here to the learning and behavioural disorder patterns of children with severe mental retardation.

SPECIFIC LEARNING DISORDERS

Specific learning disorders can exist in children who have an established neurological disorder. Many neurological disorders, for instance muscular dystrophy and spina bifida, are associated with a high incidence of learning difficulties and mental retardation. However, some of these children have an overall normal intelligence but are known to have co-existent specific learning difficulties. The severity of the learning disorders is often not directly related to the degree of physical handicap. Certain of the neurological disorders associated with particular learning difficulties, e.g. children with even mild cerebral palsy, may have a significant visuo-spatial impairment, and boys with muscular dystrophy often have expressive difficulty.

The limitations imposed by disability restricts the exploration of the environment by the young physically handicapped child. These children therefore have far less experience of their environment than the normal child. This must be taken into account in any assessment. It is important to have a knowledge of the association of certain specific learning disorders with definite neurological disorders so that such problems can be anticipated and care taken to minimise their effects as much as possible.

The other group of children who present with specific learning problems are those who have overall normal intelligence and a lack of physical disease, but are recognised, particularly when they enter formal education, as having specific learning difficulties. These children need a full multidisciplinary assessment. Taking a thorough medical history should be supplemented by an equally thorough examination. Any gross evidence of poor neuromuscular co-ordination is actively sought and satisfactory tests of hearing and vision must be undertaken. Careful psychometric analysis by an experienced psychologist is always important and a careful language assessment by a speech therapist is often useful. Observations by a physiotherapist should reveal any abnormalities of large movement and general body orientation, while an occupational therapist will be able to assess the finer movements, particularly in the hands. All such assessments should be supported by reports from teachers, nursery nurses, or health visitors as appropriate.

Children with specific learning disorders may also have symptoms that include headaches, dizziness, and abdominal symptoms—often as a secondary behavioural or emotional phenomenon.

Specific learning disorders can be divided into several groups based on the problem that is experienced by the child.

DISORDERS OF PERCEPTUAL MOTOR FUNCTION

Perceptual motor function can reasonably be expected to depend on sensory perception and the ability of the brain to receive that information. The left hemisphere of the brain is associated with the organisation of movement and the right with organisation of spatial perception. In some, hemisphere loss or damage can result in poor co-ordination between motor and sensory function. Children who are known to have a brain abnormality may show disorders of perceptual motor function. However, in most cases there is no known brain abnormality and speculation exists as to whether there is an underlying developmental delay or deficit in a part of the brain.

The clumsy child

The clumsy child is a particular example of a disorder of perceptual motor function. The typical history is of a child who is continually bumping into objects, falling down, poor at fine manipulative tasks such as doing up buttons and shoe laces, generally slow at dressing—getting clothes on back to front—often dropping objects, very poor at ball games, and generally ungainly with walking and running. This is the typical history, but often it will become obscured by superimposed emotional and behavioural disorders. The child becomes aware that these problems exist and make him less able to cope with the environment than his peers. At school this may cause a short attention span, poor concentration, poor handwriting, and marked overactivity. Examination will confirm difficulty with fine manipulative activities.

The aetiological factors of this condition—often referred to unhelpfully as *minimal brain dysfunction*—are controversial. In a few there appears to be some genetic predispositions to clumsiness. On the other hand, review of the pregnancy and perinatal histories of clumsy children do suggest a higher than usual incidence of antenatal and perinatal problems.

Early recognition is the most important aspect of management. It has been suggested that this type of motor dysfunction should be actively sought at the time of school entry. Early recognition of clumsiness in its varying forms enables specific remedial programmes to be implemented which may help avoid the experience of repeated failure at tasks which clumsy children find so much more difficult than others. The aim should be to prevent the secondary emotional and behavioural disorders that all too often accompany the situation if it goes unrecognised.

SPEECH AND LANGUAGE DISORDERS

The age of acquisition of meaningful expressive language varies greatly—from soon after one year to two and a half years in a child of normal intelligence. *Receptive language*, or comprehension, will significantly precede speech.

There are several recognised patterns of speech delay. The range may be from a persistence of infantile speech patterns with poor articulation but normal comprehension, or an apparent inability to comprehend speech due to a central brain dysfunction, to an inability to decode incoming auditory stimuli. However, the commonest cause of delayed or absent speech development will be a general delay in intellectual development. In clinical practice speech delay may be one of the commonest presentations of developmental delay.

Deafness is the second largest cause of speech and language disorders. Severe cerebral palsy, particularly spastic quadriparesis and dyskinetic cerebral palsy, is often associated with a speech and language disorder. In addition, children with severe physical handicap may suffer, as already described, from a degree of 'deprivation' such that language development may be markedly impaired. Language development will be impaired even in a normal child who suffers social deprivation. As part of the surveillance of the development of all children, patterns of speech development are carefully monitored. The early recognition of delay is important along with investigations as to its cause. It is especially important as speech delay may be an indicator of an underlying treatable condition.

Infantile autism

This may first be suspected because of a delay in developing speech. One of the major features of this condition is severe speech and language dysfunction coupled with odd mannerisms, fixed habits, and a withdrawal of the child from the environment into a world of his own. The understanding of the cause of infantile autism is uncertain. Severe deprivation, visual handicap, and deafness have all been implicated. An autistic syndrome is sometimes seen in the second or third year of life in children who are already developmentally delayed and in whom a marked regression of function may then be observed that can mimic a neurodegenerative disorder.

The loss of already acquired speech is particularly worrying and should be fully investigated. This can occur secondary to a major emotional trauma (elective mutism), cerebral degenerative disorders, a focal brain tumour, a physical brain injury to the dominant hemisphere, or very rarely in a child who has temporal lobe seizures.

Thus the evaluation of a child with a speech or language disorder has to take in a wide range of diagnostic possibilities with the need for careful multidisciplinary assessment, often over a period of time, and, equally, multidisciplinary management and education, often in a special unit.

Reading retardation

Isolated reading difficulties are all too often referred to as *dyslexia* or *word blindness*. These terms are too often applied to children who have learning difficulties that are by no means restricted to reading. More recently it has been possible to refer to a group of dyslexic disorders, in each of which a different mechanism for the reading difficulty has been postulated. Any child presenting with a severe reading disorder requires careful evaluation.

BEHAVIOURAL DISORDERS

The hyperactive child

Mention has already been made of a hyperkinetic syndrome developing in a child with unrecognised motor perceptual disorders—the clumsy child. It may also occur in a number of mentally retarded children; in children with epilepsy, particularly if treated with certain anticonvulsants, e.g. phenobarbitone; and in children of normal intelligence.

The marked restlessness, easy distractability, and short attention span associated with the hyperactivity grossly impair learning processes. The cause is uncertain in those cases not apparently associated with other disorders. The paradoxical reaction that these children show to drugs is of interest. With a number of sedative drugs their hyperactivity is significantly increased, whereas stimulant drugs from the amphetamine group decrease their overactivity. Whatever the explanation for this the use of amphetamines can be therapeutically beneficial when coupled with structured teaching programmes that are often in a one to one ratio. The outlook for the hyperkinetic child of normal intelligence is generally favourable with early active management.

The most important factor associated with behavioural disorders is the great difficulty experienced in making an accurate diagnosis.

The presence of a co-existent neurological abnormality may make it easier to understand the development of the behavioural disorder. Such understanding does not necessarily make it easier to treat.

Behavioural disorders may often require management by a child psychiatrist, even in the presence of a neurological abnormality.

For children with learning disorders, often with secondary emotional and behavioural disorders, generalisations are not appropriate. Continuing liaison between different professionals involved with such children should prevent a deficit becoming a disability, and a disability becoming a handicap.

FURTHER READING

Espir, M. L. E. and Rose, C. F. (1980). *The Basic Neurology of Speech*, 3rd edition. Blackwell Scientific Publications Limited, Oxford.

Gordon, N. and McKinely, I. (1980). *Helping the Clumsy Child*. Blackwell Scientific Publications Limited, Oxford.

Holt, K. (1977). *Developmental Paediatrics*. Volume in the Postgraduate Paediatric Series (General editor, Apley, J.). Butterworths, London.

20. Parents and professionals

In the management of most neurological disorders a team approach is essential. A very high proportion of children with neurological conditions have disorders that are, or are potentially, handicapping.

Many of these children have long-term chronic illnesses, some associated with steady deterioration in motor and intellectual function. Others are severely handicapped from birth. The care of such children must be closely associated with provision of care and support for the whole family. Such care can only be adequately provided when the professionals involved are able to work together, each complementing the other yet aiming towards the same goals.

This book contains many examples of the needs and importance of good and complementary relationships between different professional groups. If the needs of a particular child and his family are to be met as in epilepsy, severe mental retardation, cerebral palsy, neuromuscular disorders, learning disorders, structural disorders of the nervous system, and neurodegenerative disorders, then multidisciplinary management has to be meaningful.

Undoubtedly there is a role for all the health care professionals in the general management of children with neurological disorders. However, the roles that are played do not always relate to the precise professional designation of the individuals. The ability of the various professionals to complement each other is highly important in offering care. The professional boundaries must not be allowed to impinge on the concept of multidisciplinary or multiprofessional management.

Arguments over 'professional' roles are of secondary

importance to the consideration of parental roles. A fundamental argument may be as to whether there is a need for any active involvement of a particular professional worker. In the case of a child with, for example, a major physical problem the **parents should be regarded as the principal therapists**. All too often enthusiastic and dedicated therapists have unconsciously assumed parental rights. It is the responsibility of the therapist initially to assess the problems presented by the child, then to assess the therapy relevant to the child's needs, and finally to enable the parents to embark upon continuing assessment, treatment, and monitoring of their own child.

A starting point for parents is the provision for them of complete and intelligible information, both verbal and written. At an early stage opportunity should be given for questions to be asked by the parents about their child's therapy. The opportunity to meet other parents whose children appear to have similar problems may be beneficial.

A partnership must be developed between parents and professionals. This is essential for the management of children with neurological disorders—each has much to learn from the other. The tendency to 'take over' a child should be avoided and instead be replaced by the desire to provide each parent with the means to be a major therapist in the management of their child's problems—thus Mrs Smith should become John Smith's expert therapist. As therapists (and here the author includes doctors and nurses) we must avoid the risk of insinuating ourselves between parent and child and recognise that we are but advisers. For a child with a severe neurological disorder we may recognise the value of intermittent short-term residential care, but at the same time we must be sensitive to the reactions and feelings that parents may have towards other people caring for their children.

Where parental expectations of assessment may be unreal, our professional offer of support by medical, social and educational means must always include care, support and sensitivity to their own needs as well as their children.

FURTHER READING

Apley, J. (1978). *Care of the Handicapped Child. A Festschrift for Ronald McKeith.* Spastics International Medical Publications. Clinics in Developmental Medicine No 67. William Heinemann Medical Books Ltd, London.

Craft, M. (Ed) (1979). *Tredgold's Mental Retardation*, 12th edition. Baillière Tindall, London.

Drillien, C. M. and Drummond, M. B. (1978). *Neurodevelopmental Problems in Early Childhood.* Blackwell Scientific Publications Limited, Oxford.

Kirman, B. and Bicknell, J. (1975). *Mental Handicap.* Churchill Livingstone, Edinburgh.

MacKay, R. I. (1976). *Mental Handicap in Child Health Practice.* Volume in the Postgraduate Paediatric Series (General editor, Apley, J.). Butterworths, London.

Mitchell, R. G. (Ed) (1976). *Child Health in the Community.* Churchill Livingstone, Edinburgh.

Useful organisations

The following is a selection of Associations who may provide help, advice and information.

Association for all Speech Impaired Children (AFASIC)
347 Central Markets, Smithfield
London EC1A 9NM

Association for Spina Bifida and Hydrocephalus (ASBAH)
Tavistock House North
Tavistock Square, London WC1H 9HJ

Association to Combat Huntington's Chorea
Lyndhurst, Lower Hampton Road
Sunbury-on-Thames, Middlesex

British Epilepsy Association
Crowthorne House, Bigshotte
New Wokingham Road, Wokingham RG11 3AY

British Tay-Sachs Foundation
The Hospital for Sick Children
Great Ormond Street, London WC1N 3JH

Down's Children's Association
Quinborne Community Centre
Ridgacre Road, Quinton
Birmingham B32 2TW

Friedreich's Ataxia Group
12c Worplesdon Road
Guildford GV2 6RW

Hyperactive Children's Support Group
59 Meadowside, Angmering
West Sussex BN16 4BW

Migraine Trust
45 Great Ormond Street
London WC1N 3HD

The Muscular Dystrophy Group of Great Britain
Nattrass House
35 Macaulay Road, London SW4 0QP

National Association for Mental Health (MIND)
22 Harley Street
London W1N 2ED

National Society for Mentally Handicapped Children
117–123 Golden Lane
London EC1Y 0RT

Spastics Society
12 Park Crescent
London W1N 4EQ

Tuberous Sclerosis Association of Great Britain
c/o Church Farm House, Church Road
North Leigh, Oxfordshire OX8 6TX

Disabled Living Foundation
346 Kensington High Street
London W14 8NS

Royal Association for Disability and Rehabilitation (RADAR)
25 Mortimer Street
London W1N 8AB

Riding for the Disabled Association
Avenue R, National Agricultural Centre
Kenilworth, Warwickshire CV8 2LY

Toy Libraries Association
Seabrook House, Wyllyotts Manor
Darkes Lane, Potters Bar EN6 2HL

Committee on Sexual Problems of the Disabled (SPOD)
The Diorama, 14 Peto Place
London NW1 4DT

General reading list

Swaiman, K. F. and Wright, F. S. (1975). *The Practice of Paediatric Neurology.* C. V. Mosby Co, St Louis.

Menkes, J. H. (1980). *Textbook of Child Neurology,* 2nd edition. Lea and Febiger, Philadelphia.

Walton, J. N. (Ed) (1977). *Brain's Diseases of the Nervous System,* 8th edition. Oxford University Press, Oxford.

Walton, J. N. (Ed) (1974). *Disorders of Voluntary Muscle,* 3rd edition. Churchill Livingstone, Edinburgh.

Craft, M. (Ed) (1979). *Tredgold's Mental Retardation,* 12th edition. Bailliere Tindall, London.

Kirman, B. and Bicknell, J. (1975). *Mental Handicap.* Churchill Livingstone, Edinburgh.

Downie, P. A. (Ed) (1982). *Cash's Neurology for Physiotherapists,* 3rd edition. Faber and Faber, London and Boston.

Bondo, U. (1980). *Ida: Life with my Handicapped Child.* Faber and Faber, London and Boston.

Index